THE COMPLETE
Style
Guide

THE COMPLETE
Style
Guide

from the

Color Me
Beautiful
Organisation

Mary Spillane

PIATKUS

To my terrific team of CMB Consultants working throughout
Europe, Africa, the Middle East, Australia and New Zealand
helping women develop more confidence through their image.

@ 1991 Mary Spillane
CMB is registered trademark of
Color Me Beautiful Inc.

First published in 1991 by
Judy Piatkus (Publishers) Ltd
5 Windmill Street, London W1P 1HF

Reprinted 1991 (twice), 1992, 1993, 1994, 1995

**The moral right of the author
has been asserted**

*A catalogue record for this book is
available from the British Library*

ISBN 0-7499-1112-3 (Pbk)

Designed by Paul Saunders
Fashion illustrations by Lynne Robinson
Line drawing by Paul Saunders
Photography for chapters 3 and 5 by Ian Philpott
Photography for page 111 by Phil Dodd
Photography for page 99 by
Karena Perronet-Miller, courtesy
Cosmopolitan (UK)

*All colours are subject to the limitations
of the printing process*

Typeset in ITC Garamond by
Wyvern Typesetting Ltd, Bristol
Reproduction by Tenon & Polert, Hong Kong
Printed and bound in Great Britain by
The Bath Press, Avon

Contents

Acknowledgements

THIS book is the result of inspiration and work from a lot of people besides myself.

In addition to all the wonderful clients I have had the delight to work with I have also learned much from my own consultants over the years. I am especially indebted to Veronique Henderson who worked until she was mauve in the face to rationalise all the colours in our new Seasonal Palettes and convince many prestigious design houses to let us share their photographs. Liz Baker, our indefatigable PR, organised the wonderful clothes from Selfridges and Liberty used for our models. CMB trainers, Pam Howard and Madge Campbell, provided helpful advice in the drafting stages. Trevor Castleton made sure the business carried on in my absence keeping staff, consultants and clients happy. And Sue Abbott, my right arm since 1984, can quote this book chapter and verse having typed endless revisions until we got it right.

Special thanks to my consultant models: Anna Bourgeois, Sylvia Jordan, Teoh Berry, Debra Coffman, Harriet Walters, Carolyn Patrick and Sarah Wright and the generosity of Ruth Block, Diana Tanaka, Joanna Hadnutt, Lisa Pope, Sue Simmons, Jane Pringle, Michele Morgan, Christina Pardul and Amrita Ganguly who also appear in the book. Gary and Keith Beer of The Cutting Company (at Holmes Place Health Club, London SW10) are CMB's favourite hairdressers and are responsible for everyone looking so wonderful. Mary Rose Cooney of Hans Stepper UK receives special thanks for the splendid photographs showing women how eyewear can transform their image. Also thanks to all the following for the use of photographs: Armani, Elida Gibbs Ltd, Episode, Country Casuals, Fink Modelle, Jaeger, L'Oreal, Maxmara, Monsoon, Next, Paul Costelloe, Planet, Trader for Kids at Debenhams, Viyella, Windsmoor.

Judy Piatkus and her team at Piatkus Books are credited with recognising the potential for Color Me Beautiful whilst other publishers dismissed it as an American phenomenon. Gill Cormode's constructive, as well as creative editorial direction is evident throughout the book. She deserves special thanks for teaching me invaluable lessons as a first time author. My frantic pen may never stop.

Steve DiAntonio, President of CMB Inc. (USA) understood the need for us to write a book on style emanating from Europe and has enthusiastically endorsed our efforts.

My husband, Roger Luscombe, deserves credit for being so supportive during the frantic months of writing and preparation. And finally Anna and Lucy get their mummy back to play with on weekends.

Introduction

THIS book is all about you and your image. This includes everything to do with your appearance – not simply how you look but also how you act and react to other people and situations. We will work together throughout the book to see that you are making the most of yourself. We'll consider how you might look even better, be more confident, more *you* in the future, using Color Me Beautiful techniques.

Color Me Beautiful (CMB) Image Consultants work with millions of women around the world: women on large and small budgets; mothers whether at home or working; students, executives and politicians; nuns and actresses; artists, athletes and the handicapped. The last two decades have taught *all* women that they need not take second place to anyone, that they matter in their own right – and that their image is important.

I have been directing the Color Me Beautiful organisation (we use the American spelling of colour) in Britain and Europe since 1983, and these have been very exciting and rewarding years. It is thrilling to see what transformations can be achieved. Everyone can look beautiful – you just need to know how to do it.

The Complete Style Guide from the Color Me Beautiful Organisation is a synthesis of our work: the creative techniques we have developed within the CMB network, aided by interaction with many other experts in beauty, fashion, personal development and communication, who have tutored as well as worked with Color Me Beautiful. I now want to share with you these simple but effective techniques that have helped so many women to look and feel more attractive and confident. This information I pass on out of a genuine love of women, an admiration for their personal courage and an unqualified conviction that our methods really do work wonders.

Whatever your colouring, you will find that there is one palette of Seasonal Colours that really is best for you. This will contain the most flattering colours you can wear. Further, depending on the particular features of your body shape, certain styles, fabrics, designs and accessories will also be more flattering than others. But that does not mean you will become a stereotype. There will still be lots of room for an individual interpretation of your colour and style guidelines, to ensure that your best image truly reflects who you are as well as who you want to be.

THE COLOR ME BEAUTIFUL REVOLUTION

When *Color Me Beautiful* by Carole Jackson was first published in 1980, it revolutionised the way millions of women think about themselves and how they subsequently behave as consumers. It urged us to stop being influenced solely by what colours were pronounced to be 'in fashion', and to select clothes according to a colour palette that complements our own natural skin tone, eye and hair colour – because the right colours help us look healthier, more attractive, and younger. For women around the world – and over 20 million have read *Color Me Beautiful* – this made good sense. It made even better sense when they put the theory to the test. It classes people as either Spring, Summer, Autumn or Winter types, each with their own palette of flattering colours. Once you discover your season and wear clothes and make-up in your palette colours, you look better – your eyes seem brighter, your skin smoother – you simply glow.

Looking better is not the only benefit; you also save money. Your wardrobe begins to co-ordinate more successfully. All the blouses work with whatever jacket or skirt you put with them. You no longer need black, blue *and* brown shoes – just one set of neutrals that work with everything will do.

Each seasonal palette also allows you to create many outfits from fewer clothes, so you can buy better quality – knowing that the investment will go on working for you for several years. No longer need you contemplate years of trial and error and wasted expense. No longer will your wardrobes and drawers be cluttered with unwearable clothes and unused make-up. Just think what all this is going to do for your confidence and your image!

Convincing the Retailers

Colour analysed clients in the mid-80s created havoc for retailers. Although we advised our clients that their seasonal palette represented thousands of colours, and was therefore only a guide to their best colours, they had an almost evangelical zeal about their best pinks, blues, yellows and greens and would not accept alternatives, particularly from some uninitiated sales assistant perplexed by the idea that a person *could* be something called a 'spring'.

Since then, we have worked closely with the retailers to avoid such frustrations. Even hardened sceptics with long tenures in the fashion world now appreciate that the seasonal colour system is not only good for their customers but actually an incredible sales tool.

Leading cosmetic companies have also learned the benefits of guiding customers to the cool or warm part of their ranges, and special cosmetic lines have been developed, not only by Color Me Beautiful but by many other companies.

The Total Image Consultants

The success of *Color Me Beautiful* spawned a new industry known as image consulting. Today, there are some 50,000 image consultants in America alone, with several dozen good organisations operating throughout Europe. Color Me Beautiful has over 2,000 consultants worldwide, including 250 in the UK and 400 in Europe.

Once people had had their colours analysed they wanted to know still more – about what style of clothes suited them, how to update their wardrobe on a limited budget, how to dress appropriately for different occasions, how to put together a business wardrobe, how to look fashionable whatever their age – the list goes on and on. In response, CMB extended its expertise and developed a range of services, or programmes, which are available through our specially trained network of consultants (see below). You, too, are about to benefit from all this expertise.

CMB PROGRAMMES

For Women
Personal Colour Analysis
Make-Up Techniques
Personal Style
Wardrobe Planning
Personal Shopping
Fashion Updates
Bridal Consultations
How to Dress the Man in Your Life
Facial Fitness Exercises
Skin Care Clinics

For Men
Personal Colour Analysis
Style Assessments
Wardrobe Planning
Travel and Packing Ideas
Personal Shopping

For Schools
Importance of Image Presentations
Personal Grooming
Colour and Style Clinics

For Companies
Professional Image Seminars
Media Training
Body Language
Etiquette

For Retailers
Customer Service using CMB
    Colour and Style Techniques
In-Store Promotions and Workshops

YOUR COMPLETE STYLE GUIDE

The Complete Style Guide from the Color Me Beautiful Organisation gives valuable new information on colour and style for women of all walks of life and of all ages. You'll learn not only what colours make you look good but what colours make you feel good. You'll find out what physical assets you might be hiding and how to make the most of what you've got – whatever your figure shape or size.

The colour palettes have also been made even simpler to use. This was in response to requests from women who felt they did not quite fit into any one of the original four seasons. There are now three palettes for each season, making 12 possible seasonal types: Spring types may be Light, Warm or Clear; Summer types may be Light, Cool or Soft; Autumns may be Soft, Warm or Deep; and Winters may be Deep, Cool or Clear. This may sound more complicated, but I guarantee it's not! And whether you are new to Color Me Beautiful or familiar with our techniques, in Chapter 3 I show you how to discover which of the 12 seasonal types you are using a quick and foolproof method. I will then show you how to use this valuable knowledge to choose your most flattering colours to wear for clothes and make-up.

And do you know that you have vitamins in your wardrobe? I'm referring to 11 key colours that can boost your success depending on the occasion. In Chapter 4 you'll learn the power of each and how to maximise their effect.

The finishing touches you give your look can make or break your image and I give make-up and personal grooming tips in Chapter 6. I also give advice on choosing glasses, whether sunglasses or prescription ones. This is something we are repeatedly asked for at Color Me Beautiful: how *do* you choose flattering frames? All will be revealed.

Hair should be your crowning glory, so follow the advice in Chapter 6 on choosing a hairstyle to suit not only your hair type and face shape, but also your lifestyle. And if you do colour your hair, learn some very important guidelines on choosing a colour to suit your Season – a colour that won't look unnatural or harsh.

Do you have a style personality? Would you like to develop one? Recognising your own personal style preferences will help you to find the clothes that make you feel most comfortable and most *you*. Chapter 7 will show you how. It will also help you create a harmonious wardrobe rather than a muddle of contradictory styles that could never work together, saving you time and money.

Since many of you are women who work part-time or full-time outside the home, this book focuses much of its attention on your concerns for getting ahead and earning the recognition you deserve. Chapter 8 is full of image tips for every stage of your career. In Chapter 9 you'll discover how to put together a successful and practical working wardrobe depending on what line of work you are in.

We have much to learn from each other, and other cultures. Different nationalities project different images from our own. In Chapter 10 you'll learn how to develop international chic and there are useful tips for travelling abroad.

The last two chapters in the book deal with two important aspects of your body: its language and its health. Both are vital to your style and image, so learn how to make the most of yours.

Now let's begin.

chapter one

Does *image matter?*

TODAY'S concern with appearance is more pervasive at every level of Western society than it was even 30 years ago. There are three main reasons. Firstly, we have increased mobility – most of us move home and change jobs more frequently than our parents did and as a result are continually having to re-establish our identities with new people in new environments. Secondly, there is the impact of television – it has made us very judgemental of visual images and what they mean. Thirdly, there is the changing role of women, many of whom now defy traditional stereotyping and are seen in new and challenging roles. Let's consider these three factors in a little more detail.

Moving On

Do you still live in the same neighbourhood where you grew up? Or have you moved house or jobs more than once in the last 10 years? Moving house and changing jobs are two of the most stressful life experiences, because when we move we leave our history behind and have to start all over again. We have to convince new neighbours, employers and acquaintances that we are worth knowing, that we are trustworthy, friendly, creative or whatever we know ourselves to be and want others to believe.

Until our new contacts get to know us, they will judge us by our appearance and our behaviour. The trappings of our lifestyle 'explain' a lot before we have a chance to elaborate for ourselves. The car we drive, where we live, how we decorate our homes, how our children behave, where they attend school, the clothes we wear, the food we eat, what we drink – all help to complete the portrait. The stark reality is that image matters.

In such circumstances, projecting a positive image helps us not only to succeed but also to fit into the new organisation as quickly as possible. No one likes to be an outsider; we all strive for acceptance. In this book we shall look at how your working image can catapult you forward or perhaps hold you back in your career. You will discover why it is important to earn the recognition and remuneration you deserve, why you should value yourself more. When you project an image that signals 'I value myself', others can't help treating you the same.

Our 30-Second Culture

Television has had a profound effect on all of us not only because we increasingly spend more time viewing it, but because it has developed our abilities to form judgements in all things visual. After a lifetime of being bombarded with 10 to 30 second advertisements in which messages are clearly and persuasively conveyed through imagery, we are programmed to give all people and things a fleeting 'size-up' during which we decide to hire or not to hire, to respect or not to respect, to buy or not to buy.

In the 1970s, Professor Albert Mehrabian's study *Silent Messages* proved convincingly that visual images matter a lot. He found that the impact we make on each other depends: 55% on how we look and behave; 38% on how we speak and 7% on what we say. Whether we like it or not, that's the way it is.

I share these statistics with all my clients, whatever their lifestyle or vocation, to prove just how important your image is, and the value people place on first impressions. If your image conflicts with your message you'll have a herculean task getting the right message across. If you expect anyone to believe you're successful, creative, approachable or whatever, your image must say this before you even open your mouth.

Television, rightly or wrongly, has made us all 'expert' image analysts. It also creates role models, for style as well as behaviour. During the 1980s the thriving, thrusting glitzy gals of American soap operas like *Dallas* and *Dynasty* spurred women around the world to artificially extend their shoulders with formidable pads, and to don 'power suits'. The designs may have first appeared on exclusive catwalks in Paris, but the TV soap queens made them accessible and desirable to the masses. In the 1990s, we are looking more closely at how our attitudes (and those of men) are being conditioned, even manipulated, by the media. We have become older, wiser and, hopefully, less gullible. Advertisers are beginning to understand that we want strong, positive but also realistic images of ourselves. Even so, we still pass split second judgements on others, as they do upon us, based purely on image – how we/they look and how we/they act.

New Roles – New Challenges

Young women today have terrific role models in others who have chosen a family life, a career or are juggling both. Our lives are becoming ever more diverse. Books and magazines of varying style, political bent and feminist view compete for our attention. And the varied roles we assume are also mirrored in television and film drama. Now, women are portrayed as leaders, policewomen, detectives, lawyers, investment bankers, soldiers and doctors, as well as daughters, wives and mistresses.

So, advice and role models abound. But if you are vying for a promotion in your chosen career, it is smart to start dressing as if it had already happened. To look authoritative and confident you don't need to dress like a pseudo-male in a severely tailored suit or wear drab unflattering colours. The challenge is to assess what the expectations are likely to be and then look and act the part in a way that complements you and your personality.

Your image should be neither contrived nor predictable. When you introduce yourself you want others to be impressed with *you*, the individual, first. The right image is not about expensive clothes or co-ordinated accessories, it's about being *you*, being appropriate for the roles you play and being part of today. Once you accept this, you can begin to explore how you might enhance your image in a way that's right for you.

YOUR PERSONAL VALUATION

Do you get up in the morning and look in the mirror without any emotional baggage? Most of us can't. We tend to concentrate on the features we consider 'imperfect' rather than on our good points. But why have we developed such negative self images? Are men to blame? Is it the media's fault? Or do we actually perpetuate the problem with our absurd self-consciousness?

Even at exercise clubs, where you find active women in pursuit of health and fitness, there is still a universal preoccupation with fat and personal 'shortcomings' relating to legs, bosoms, bottoms, knees, ankles, skin and hair. The litany of woes I listen to week after week in the shower room at my club, (from women who exercise three or four times a week) is deafening! Whether they be a size 6 or 16, and even when fit and trim, many women continue to despair because they still do not match up to that mythical image of perfection they are continually striving to achieve. Are men so preoccupied? I doubt it.

Life is too short for such a mindless pursuit of the unattainable. It's time to give up the fruitless pursuit of the 'perfect' body and accept your own uniqueness. Concentrate your attention on a sensible, well-balanced diet that provides you with all the nutrients you need for good health, and sufficient exercise to keep you trim, strong – and supple. Our bodies are important aesthetically, yes, but also for how well they function.

Focus your attention on the *potential* of you and your body, no matter what your size or shape. Beauty is, by definition, a quality that gives the eye or the other senses pleasure. We can please our senses by how we use colour, fabric and design. All three can be used in ways that are complimentary to *you* regardless of whether you are a size 6 or 26. When you create an image that is a true reflection of yourself we stop and notice *you*. Bringing out one's own true beauty is the challenge within the reach of each of us. So forget those images of 'beauty' in glossy magazines and on the TV, and instead look into the mirror.

Firstly I want you to appraise your assets – those physical resources that you do have. We are going to work with them, to create your very best personal image. Let's assess them now. You may be pleasantly surprised by how many ticks you can mark on the Personal Valuation chart.

MY PERSONAL VALUATION

	Definite Asset	Hidden Asset	Liability
Skin	☐	☐	☐
Hair	☐	☐	☐
Eyebrows	☐	☐	☐
Eyes	☐	☐	☐
Nose	☐	☐	☐
Mouth	☐	☐	☐
Teeth	☐	☐	☐
Smile!	☐	☐	☐
Cheekbones	☐	☐	☐
Chin/Jawline	☐	☐	☐
Neck	☐	☐	☐
Shoulders	☐	☐	☐
Bust	☐	☐	☐
Waist	☐	☐	☐
Hips	☐	☐	☐
Bottom	☐	☐	☐
Legs	☐	☐	☐
Arms	☐	☐	☐
Hands	☐	☐	☐
Feet	☐	☐	☐

Your Definite Assets

If you haven't ticked at least two Definite Assets then you have a very poor self-image indeed. I can name two of your Definite Assets without even seeing you!

Everyone's eyes are an asset. They are also unique – have you seen all the colours in your irises? No? Well, go back to the mirror and have a good look. Once you've done that, tick your eyes as a Definite Asset.

Now sit in front of the mirror. Think of the last ridiculous thing you did or the funniest situation you can remember. Have a good giggle. See your smile? It's irresistible, everyone's is. If you haven't ticked your smile as a Definite Asset go back and do so now.

For the other Definite Assets you have ticked, ask yourself if you are making the most of them. For example, if you have lovely prominent cheekbones does your hairstyle hide them or accentuate them? Do you show off your trim waistline in waist-hugging styles and attractive belts or do you hide it under too many bulky layers?

In the following chapters you'll find many useful tips for making the most of your best features.

Your Hidden Assets

A Hidden Asset is something you could be featuring more but don't know how.

Perhaps you have healthy, thick, shiny hair but tend to tie it back from your face for convenience. It could be that a well-cut, shorter style would be just as easy to manage, and emphasise the thickness and shine of your hair.

Or you may have beautifully shaped hands and long, slender fingers but neglect to manicure them – or, even worse, bite your nails.

Perhaps you've ticked off several Hidden Assets because they are quite literally 'hidden' under flab. If flab is your problem – rather than excess weight – you could easily turn those Hidden Assets into Definite Assets just by toning up. Don't sigh! I'm not going to recommend a serious aerobics schedule. You could tone up your body within weeks simply by walking briskly for a minimum of 20 minutes, three or four times a week. Also, when watching TV, stretch out on the floor and limber up your lazy limbs.

It's easy to realise your assets if you have the motivation.

Your Liabilities

It's an honest woman who's got a few of these ticked. More than five is excessive and some of those could really be Hidden Assets if only you knew what to do. As you read through the following chapters you'll learn how you can turn any Liability into an Asset. Take comfort, few of us look like mythical goddesses – and none of us remains so indefinitely. We've all got challenges that, if dealt with, can be minimised if not negated.

chapter two

New look required

MODERN women experience many phases throughout their lives. More life options and a longer lifespan mean more possibilities, more phases and more stress. Stress, we're told by the experts, is both healthy and harmful. It can make us perform better, demand more and achieve greater satisfaction. On the discount side it can push us under and into that dark abyss known as depression – which is hitting more and more women at some point in their lives.

So what does a book about image and style have to do with depression? Lots – because it can often be traced back to a poor self-image unwittingly introduced in childhood: 'You're not as pretty as your sister'; reinforced at school by 'You're too fat to be cool'. It is then perpetuated through adulthood: 'Don't wear colours; black makes you look slimmer', followed by a full blown mid-to-late life crisis, 'I'm simply past it'. Does it sound familiar?

The good news is that a new, positive image can be more therapeutic to women who are truly depressed than any mood-altering drugs. If you are happy with your image, you will respect yourself more and earn the respect you deserve from others.

Even those of us who are not depressed, and who have a fairly confident self-image, at one time or another have looked into the mirror and been shocked by our reflection. No bad thing if it motivates us to make healthy changes for the better.

The psychologist, Elizabeth Kübler Ross, developed a curve to describe the process of change. If we relate this change curve to your image development, at what stage are you at the moment?

Stage 1: SHOCK   Do I really look like that? What happened to my skin, my waist, my legs?

Stage 2: DENIAL   I'm just being silly – I don't look so bad. People will just have to take me for who I am.

Stage 3: FRUSTRATION   My wardrobe is full of clothes but I have nothing to wear. What on earth is fashion all about these days? Why do I look so tired, so pale? Nothing suits me.

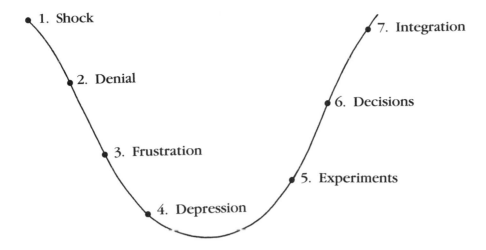

1. Shock
2. Denial
3. Frustration
4. Depression
5. Experiments
6. Decisions
7. Integration

Stage 4: DEPRESSION   There's no hope for me. My clothes are horrible. My figure's gone, my skin is lifeless, my hair mousey. Why bother?

Stage 5: EXPERIMENTS   I don't want to look like this. Make me over, please. Turn me into someone different, someone glamorous, anyone but ME.

Stage 6: DECISIONS   What I really need is advice on what suits me – why try to look like someone else?

Stage 7: INTEGRATION   What do you think of my new hairstyle and outfit? I feel terrific yet I'm still me!

Let's explore some key life transitions. I'll use case studies of CMB clients to illustrate the importance of your appearance at such times; indeed, at any time.

TRANSITION: From Schoolgirl to Career Woman

Most young women want to stand on their own two feet financially and are keen to prove their capabilities. But how do you advance beyond the reception desk? How can you project an image that says you are capable of more?

At 21, Gina faced that dilemma. She was the cornerstone of the busy buying office of a large department store, having entered retailing from secretarial college and worked her way up from general typist to Personal Assistant to the Buyer in two years. But Gina was bored and no longer felt challenged as a P.A. She had her sights on management training but had been discouraged for silly reasons from pursuing openings that other less able secretaries had won. She knew her image wasn't perfect, but she was at the Denial stage of the image development curve. One day she marched into her boss's office and demanded to know why she wasn't management training material.

'I just had to tell her that we couldn't place her out-front, representing the company, because of how she looked,' explained Gina's boss. 'The poor girl has an hormonal imbalance which means she's very overweight and, despite her bubbly personality, she also dresses very drearily.'

But Gina persisted and the management said they'd consider her if she could improve her image. She was sent to CMB to discover what might be possible.

We discussed Gina's problems head on. I suggested that we examined her diet and exercise programme to see if she was using the medical problem as an excuse not to bother. Gina agreed that she ate too much of the wrong foods, particularly when feeling low, and promised to keep a record of everything she ate for a week, so we could see exactly where the extra calories came from. She also began walking part of the way to and from work.

Now that she had moral support Gina kept a conscientious record of her eating pattern and even though she was being more careful *because* it was all being noted down, she got quite a shock when we calculated the excess calories in just one week. She went back to her doctor for a diet sheet and a weekly weigh-in which kept her on the straight and narrow. Progress was slow but steady and Gina had an important goal to spur her on.

One more immediate improvement was that Gina learned how to wear make-up, not only to look like management material but to highlight her prettiness. A new hair style 'opened up' her face and also made her look slimmer.

Gina's weight problem had been exacerbated by the dreary styles and colours she wore. We showed her how longer jackets distracted the eye from her short waist, and dressed her in blends of one colour from head to toe for an elegant, professional and slimming result. Visually she shed half a stone.

One year later, Gina is a smart dresser, 1½ stone (9.5 kg) lighter, fitter than she has been in years – and well on her way in the management programme. She's more confident too, and planning to move into her own flat any day now.

TRANSITION: From Independent to Dependent

Many of us opt to give up careers and our own income to be a stay-at-home wife and mother, for a few months or years, or for a lifetime. And indeed, these can be two of the most fulfilling roles there are for women. But some people experience a loss of identity when they lose their independence. Their priorities include everyone and everything but themselves. Such self-sacrifice is unnecessary – and unwise! Sally had fallen into just such a Dependency Trap.

It's not surprising that Sally has previously found little time to spend on her own image and style: her two school-age sons, Toby and Sam, are always taking part in extra-curricular activities and her daughter, Lottie, is almost two years old, so virtually every minute is taken up seeing to their needs and demands. 'I just don't seem to have time to think about myself,' explained Sally. 'It's only when I catch sight of my reflection that I see how I really look and I don't like what I see! I would love to feel confident and happy with my looks again, whether I'm taking the boys to tennis coaching or going out with my husband, Keith. The trouble is that I just don't know where to start.' Sally came to CMB when she was at Stage 5 of the curve, and ready to experiment with her look.

With pregnancy now firmly behind her, Sally began working on regaining her figure. Initially, she simply made a point of doing some exercises we recommended while Lottie was taking her afternoon nap. After a few weeks she began to feel more supple and was hugely encouraged to notice that her clothes fitted more comfortably – and she had more energy.

Sally's other big hang-up was that she hadn't any idea how to choose clothes to suit her. We helped her to discover her Soft Autumn palette and advised her on styles to flatter her figure immediately. Later, Sally said, 'I truly feel made over. In fact, I bumped into several people in the supermarket last week who actually said I looked glamorous! It's proved to me that I can look good whatever I'm doing and without spending hours in front of the mirror!'

TRANSITION: From Working Woman to Retiree

No one approaches the end of their career without some trepidation. We know we should look forward to retirement as a time to pursue neglected hobbies as well as new interests, and to spend more time with friends and family. But this is a pretty dramatic life change if not planned for in advance.

Increasingly, women in their late 50s and 60s are becoming less resigned to 'growing old gracefully.' And that is real progress. Whatever her age, every woman's image is very much linked to her confidence and self-esteem; no one is or should ever feel 'past it' or 'over the hill.' At any age you can be up-to-date in your outlook and style. Being current or 'with it' at 60 isn't the same as when you were 20, of course, but there's no reason not to have fun with colour and fashions simply because you are ageing.

Julie didn't want to give up her well-paid, prestigious job as a senior secretary at 58 but was pressured into doing so. Her husband had already retired and wanted her companionship; her daughter needed her to watch the grandchildren while she studied for her nursing qualification. Julie didn't 'have to' work and just 'wanting to' wasn't a good enough reason for her family.

'As my last day at work drew near I felt worse by the minute. The prospect of being at home every day rather than going to the office terrified me.'

To reassure herself, Julie decided to attend a colour analysis session but didn't tell anyone. She didn't want any chiding about being too old to worry about how she looked. The session proved to be the booster she needed.

'The consultant showed me how to use more colour and to have some fun with shades I'd never considered before. That was two years ago, and one of the best investments I've ever made. I bother every day with how I look and get compliments from strangers as well as my grandchildren. Now that my daughter is well on her way to qualifying as a nurse I'm also back working part-time. At 60 they've offered me a full-time job but I've decided to stay part-time to ease into retirement. Winding down my career seems so much easier now, because I still feel good about myself and how I look.'

I hope that this brief introduction to three very different women – each from a different generation and with their own individual viewpoint and priorities, but united in a desire to do something positive about their image and style – will inspire *you*. In the following chapter we will take a close look at that all-important factor: the colour in your life.

chapter three

Discover your colours

COLOUR Analysis is simply a careful assessment of your natural colouring – of eyes, skin and hair – in order to determine what colours for clothes and make-up are most complimentary for you. Most of us have always felt some colours suited us rather better than others, but it was all a matter of experimentation, trial and error – until the Color Me Beautiful Organisation introduced the Seasonal Colour Palette. It had a wonderful sense of logic: just analyse your natural colouring and then wear the relevant palette of Spring, Summer, Autumn or Winter to look wonderful. When your clothes and make-up complement your colouring you look natural and exciting. In your right colours we notice you first; your clothes become an afterthought.

Each Seasonal Colour Palette shows sample colours that are best for women of that type. But these are only guides to the countless possibilities that appear every year, thanks to the new dyes used in fashion. Once you know your Season it is easy to develop a wardrobe that co-ordinates since the colours within each palette are harmonious and all work together beautifully.

Millions of women who've adopted the system can confirm that it is not limiting but liberating. They have learned how to complement not negate their natural colouring so they look so much better: healthier, more attractive and confident. No longer do they suffer the frustrations of shopping without knowing what suits them, of buying things that are wrong or don't go with anything else they have and just hang around cluttering their wardrobes. Colour analysed women have wardrobes that work *for* them, not against them.

HOW 'COLOUR-CONSCIOUS' ARE YOU?

Before I explain the different Seasonal Colour Palettes and how we've expanded them to give you even more possibilities of looking wonderful and saving money, I want you to reflect first on your own approach to colour. No doubt you have some terrific items in your wardrobe that make you look and feel super. But then there are a few things that when you've worn them you haven't felt so confident or good. Next to these questionable clothes are the known disasters, perhaps items bought on impulse. No amount of make-up seems to compensate for the effect of their unflattering shade.

To find out how colour-conscious you are and if you are shopping wisely, answer the following questions.

1. When you open the wardrobe do you see many colours of the rainbow?

2. Are there some colours that make you look pale, and that always require more make-up?

3. When you wear black do you notice the clothes more than your face? (Get an honest friend to advise you.)

4. Do you have both pure white and ivory blouses?

5. Do you have black and brown as well as navy-blue shoes?

6. With your suits do you always wear the same blouses, producing the same colour combinations?

7. Do you have warm-toned lipsticks, such as peach and terracotta, as well as cool-toned lipsticks, such as fuchsia and plum?

8. Do you stick to the same few colours because you know they work?

9. Do you have clothes in royal blue as well as pastel blue or grey blue?

10. Do you wear one lipstick with everything?

Results

If you answered 'Yes' to a maximum of two questions, you have a good idea about what suits you and may only need some fine-tuning with your colours.

If you answered 'Yes' to three to six questions, you are confused and wasting a lot of money.

If you answered 'Yes' to seven or more questions, you are pouring money down the drain and not making the most of your natural good looks. So read on!

THE SEASONAL COLOUR SYSTEM FINE-TUNED

CMB have colour analysed millions of women and men since 1980. And with the feedback of over 2,000 of our image consultants testing colours around the world, certain patterns emerged when we were applying the Seasonal Colours. For example, not all Spring types are alike. Some are light and delicate, others are quite golden with some having very dark hair. We always had to qualify our advice for each client, telling her which of her seasonal colours were best to wear near her face and which were better to be mixed in prints or used in moderation. Experience showed us that often people didn't fit neatly into one Season – although one particular Season would be best for a person's neutrals and her basic colours and make-up, she could also wear a complementary group from another season.

The Colour Notation System

Perhaps the greatest influence on fine-tuning CMB's colour analysis has been the Colour Notation system developed by Albert Munsell, a 19th Century artist from Boston, Massachussetts. He defined colours and their relationship of Hue, Value and Chroma. Before the fine-tuning, colour analysis focused on just two aspects of a person's colouring: the Hue (how cool or warm they appeared) and the Value (how light or dark they were).

But there are people who don't immediately appear as either cool or warm. They might also not be strikingly light or dark. Instead some have a soft, muted look, like many Autumns and Summers. Others strike us as predominantly bright or clear, with clear jewel-like eyes, like many Springs and Winters. Where did these women fit in? Clearly, we needed to hone further the Seasonal Palettes, to provide all women with a better understanding of how to use their colours.

The original Seasonal Colour system omitted one key element of Munsell's analysis: Chroma, that is, how Clear or Muted a person's colouring appeared. In the early 1980s, Doris Pooser, then a CMB Consultant in the Far East, put forward an interpretation of the seasonal system incorporating Hue, Value, and Chroma in her book, entitled *Always In Style*. That occasioned the fine-tuning! CMB had also discovered that there were three distinct types within each Season. Rather than just tell someone she was an Autumn, for example, we were now able to clarify what *type* of Autumn. If she was a soft muted type we would refer to her as a Soft Autumn. This type can blend in a few colours from the Summer palette successfully and should avoid the more golden colours from the original, basic Autumn season. If she was a warm golden Autumn, we would refer to her as a Warm Autumn. This woman could wear some of the golden shades from the Spring palette, but she should avoid the deepest Autumn colours. If she had rich, strong Autumn colouring, then she would be classified as a Deep Autumn. The very golden shades wouldn't be too terrific on her, while the deepest end of the Autumn palette would look great. This woman could also use black and a few other colours from the Winter palette with success.

That is why, instead of just four Seasonal Palettes there are now 12: three interpretations for each Season. But don't panic! If you already know your Season you'll quickly learn how to recognise the special characteristics of your colouring and wear colour even more effectively. You may find you've been instinctively using your best colours all along. So I hope there's some confirmation along with welcome new possibilities. And if you are a newcomer to CMB and colour analysis, you can feel confident and excited that you will be able to determine your exact Seasonal Palette – the one that shows the most flattering colours that you can wear.

COLOUR ANALYSING YOURSELF: Finding Your Season

As I have already explained, the Four Seasons have been expanded to cover 12 types. Springs may be Light, Warm or Clear. Summers may be Light, Cool or

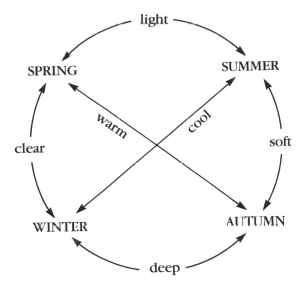

Soft. Autumns may be Soft, Warm or Deep. Winters may be Deep, Cool or Clear.

The first step in finding your seasonal type is to decide on your key colour characteristics. Using Munsell's concept, now widely recognised by colour analysts as the most accurate approach to describing colour, you'll be able to determine your predominant colour characteristics. Look at the chart on page 24 and choose which colour characteristic best describes your overall look. Try to assess your natural colouring without make-up and in natural daylight so as not to be influenced by any artificial effects. Then you'll want to determine which seasonal option gives you the widest choice of colours to be worn near your face with greatest effect. You will share many colours in common with the companion season in your key colouring characteristics. For example, both Deep Winters and Deep Autumns look terrific in black, true red, royal blue, emerald green and charcoal. But the Deep Autumn is much better in salmon pinks, terracottas and bronze tones while the Deep Winter needs her deep hot pink, blue red and bright periwinkle to really sparkle.

You might have some difficulty deciding your dominant characteristics. Perhaps your look could be interpreted in two ways. For example, someone with freckles, auburn hair and brown eyes has warm features. But she might also consider her colouring strong and rich. The task for her would be to test whether a Deep Autumn palette would be more flattering than a Warm Autumn palette. You can try different possibilities on yourself by colour draping.

COLOUR DRAPING

If you have difficulty deciding between two seasonal possibilities, colour draping is a simple way of assessing exactly which of the two you are. It involves holding blocks of colours from the two different palettes against you, and deciding which shade of a particular colour looks best. You should find that more colours from one palette will look good, and this will be your correct Seasonal Palette.

Key Colour Characteristics	Seasonal Possibilities
STRONG AND RICH	Deep Autumn or Deep Winter
LIGHT AND FAIR	Light Spring or Light Summer
WARM AND GOLDEN	Warm Spring or Warm Autumn
COOL AND ROSY	Cool Summer or Cool Winter
SOFT AND MUTED	Soft Summer or Soft Autumn
CLEAR AND BRIGHT	Clear Spring or Clear Winter

To accurately assess your colouring, choose a time when you have no make-up on, and seat yourself in front of a large mirror near a window with good natural daylight.

You'll be testing shades of different colours to see what patterns emerge. Suggestions for which colours to try are given on pages 25 to 26. Hold a large block of the suggested colour (scarves, T-shirts, sweaters, even towels, will do) under your face to see the effect. Remember, you are assessing how each looks with your particular skin, eye and hair colouring. It is important to consider the effect of the colours with your natural colouring, so if you colour your hair you will find it easier to cover it up completely for this assessment (use something off-white to cover it with) and test the colours against skin and eyes only.

You are trying to determine three things:

1. How much strength of colour you can take. Ask yourself, 'Do I wear the colour or does it wear me?'

2. If warmer tones suit you better than cooler ones. Ask yourself, 'Which are more natural looking?'

3. If contrasting colours or muted blends are more flattering. Ask yourself, 'Which look richer/more expensive?'

Then see the descriptions and palettes for each Seasonal type (on pages 34–57) for further comparison.

Strong and Rich

If this is your key colour characteristic you will be either a Deep Autumn or a Deep Winter. You will have dark hair and a rich eye colour – brown, hazel or green. You probably already know that sugary pastels make you look insignificant and will most likely prefer bold primary colours. You may have a particular preference for black.

To assess whether the warmer deep colours of Autumn are better for you than the cooler deep colours of Winter, compare the following colours near your face:

Deep Autumn		Deep Winter
Salmon Pink	vs.	Magenta
Light Peach	vs.	Icy Pink
Terracotta	vs.	Cranberry

Light and Fair

If this is your key colour characteristic, you will be either a Light Spring or a Light Summer. Fair hair, a delicate eye and light skintone best describe you. By contrast to the strong and rich colour types you probably love pastels and look elegant in soft light colours as well as medium tones. More than likely your eyes are soft blue or blue-grey

To determine if you look better with a warm light palette (Light Spring), rather than a cool light palette (Light Summer), try comparing the following colours near your face:

Light Spring		Light Summer
Bright Coral	vs.	Deep Rose
Camel	vs.	Cocoa
Light Moss	vs.	Blue Green

Warm and Golden

If you have an abundance of freckles and red, golden blonde or natural warm highlights in your hair, your key colour characteristic is probably Warm and Golden. But are you a Warm Spring or a Warm Autumn? You probably already know that fuchsia, burgundy and black don't suit you, but love yourself in many shades of gold, green and salmon.

Try comparing the following colours near your face to determine if you are a soft version (Warm Spring) or a strong version (Warm Autumn):

Warm Spring		Warm Autumn
Mango	vs.	Salmon
Medium Blue	vs.	Jade
Clear Bright Red	vs.	Bittersweet

Cool and Rosy

If you chose Cool and Rosy as your key colour characteristic, you are either a Cool Summer or a Cool Winter. You probably can't abide yourself in any shade of brown or orange and instinctively prefer rose pinks over bright coral lipsticks.

Cool women will often have grey hair with any eye colour. Your skin is a key factor and it will be neutral beige or decidedly pink in tone.

You'll want to see if a soft cool palette (Cool Summer) is better for you than a strong cool palette (Cool Winter). Compare these shades near your face:

Cool Summer		Cool Winter
Soft White	vs.	Pure White
Soft Fuchsia	vs.	Fuchsia
Blue Red	vs.	True Red

Soft and Muted

Women whose key colour characteristic is Soft and Muted will be either a Soft Summer or a Soft Autumn. They often describe their hair as mousy, their eye colour as muddy and their skin tone as neutral. If this is you, you know that bright colours make you look garish. Women in this category often have light or medium brown hair, which does benefit from highlighting. Elegant, rich colours make them look their best.

To see if you are a cool version (a Soft Summer) or a warm version (a Soft Autumn), try comparing the following colours near your face:

Soft Summer		Soft Autumn
Spruce Green	vs.	Olive Green
Soft Fuchsia	vs.	Salmon Pink
Burgundy	vs.	Mahogany

Clear and Bright

If Clear and Bright is your key colour characteristic you will be either a Clear Spring or a Clear Winter. You will have jewel-like eyes and a striking contrast between your hair, which is dark, and your skin tone, which is light. Blended or muddy colours make you look tired and even sickly. Clarity is the key. Your blues, greens, pink and reds all need to be bright, never dusty.

To see if you are a cool version (a Clear Winter) rather than a warm version (a Clear Spring), try comparing the following colours near your face:

Clear Spring		Clear Winter
Warm Pastel Pink	vs.	Fuchsia
True Green	vs.	Pine Green
True Blue	vs.	Royal Blue

ETHNIC VARIETIES

Our seasonal colour system applies to every ethnic group – but that is not to say that in every country there is an equal mix of the seasons.

In Japan, for example, where there are no natural blondes, redheads or blue-eyed people, you won't find indigenous examples of Summer and Spring types. However, there are many varieties of Autumns and Winters so, with the new expanded system presented in this book, there will still be distinctive choices.

In other Asian (such as the Indian sub-continent) and African countries, the range narrows further, with most of the native population being Deep Autumns or Deep Winters. Hence, it's no wonder that Indian saris are mainly in primary colours or rich, spicy hues. In Scandinavia, by contrast, the true Winter or Deep Autumn is rare (except among those with Finnish blood!) and there is instead an abundance of Springs, Summers and Soft Autumns.

On page 33 are four models with different ethnic looks. We chose the girls to make a particular point. They all have an obviously deep look, yet they do not possess the same key colour characteristics: Diana, Amrita and Ruth's key colour characteristics are strong and rich, and Harriet's is clear and bright. Nor do they all share the some Season: Diana favours the warm, deep colours of the Deep Autumn Palette, while Amrita and Ruth favour the cool deep colours of Deep Winter, and Harriet's clear, bright and cool look makes her a Clear Winter.

FINE-TUNING YOUR PERSONAL COLOUR ANALYSIS

You should now have a good basic idea of your key colour characteristic and may be quite sure which seasonal type is best for you. But to be absolutely sure you have considered all your possible options, let's assess your hair colour, eyes and skintone in more detail.

Hair Colour

Although all seasonal types can tint, highlight or lowlight their hair effectively (see pages 105–8), don't consider any artificial toning when analysing your type. It is important to use this guide against your *natural* hair colour.

Colour	Comment	Try
Ash blonde	Not yellow or golden	Light Summer or Light Spring
Golden blonde, strawberry blonde or red	Warm highlights	Warm Spring or Warm Autumn
Light to medium brown	Goes golden in the sun	Light Spring or Light Summer
Mousy brown	No natural highlights	Soft Summer or Soft Autumn
Medium brown	Not mousy	Clear Spring or Deep Autumn

Colour	Comment	Try
Medium to deep auburn	No blonde highlights	Deep Autumn or Deep Winter
Chestnut to dark brown	No blonde highlights	Clear Spring; Deep Autumn; Deep or Clear Winter
Dark black	Possibly with a blue cast	Clear or Deep Winter, Deep Autumn
Warm grey	Yellowish, not particularly pretty	Light or Warm Spring; Soft or Warm Autumn
Soft grey, Ash grey	Naturally attractive	Light Spring; Light or Cool Summer
Salt 'n' pepper, Silver	Terrific	Clear Spring; Winters or Cool Summer

MY NATURAL HAIR COLOUR IS _____

Eyes

Take a good close look at your eyes. What is the overall colour effect? How clear, deep or soft are they? Here are the possibilities:

Colour	Comment	Try
Clear blue, green, turquoise or bright hazel	Bright	Clear or Light Spring; Clear Winter
Grey, soft blue	Cool/Dusty	Summers
Hazel, topaz, golden brown, warm turquoise	Warm/Golden	Warm Spring or Warm Autumn
Soft hazel or turquoise	Muddy	Soft Summer, Soft Autumn
Dark brown, rich hazel	Deep	Deep Autumn or Deep Winter

MY EYE COLOUR IS _____

Skintone

Assess your overall skintone without make-up. The following comments about the effects of the sun are a helpful guide.

Colour	Comment	Try
Porcelain	Can't abide the sun	Clear Winter; Springs; Light Summer

Colour	Comment	Try
Ivory	Burn quickly in the sun, freckle or go creamy but fade fast	Springs, Summers, Soft Autumn
Pink beige	Tan fast but get a pinky cast	Light or Cool Summer; Light Spring
Neutral beige/Oriental	Tan easily but go brown not pink	Soft or Deep Autumn; Cool or Deep Winter
Warm beige/Oriental/ Asian	Some freckling but go golden brown	Autumns
Golden brown/Asian/ Latin/Black	Go bronze in the sun	Autumns or Deep Winter
Cool Brown/Asian/Latin/ Black	Go deeper, almost blue black in sun	Deep or Cool Winter
Olive/Asian/Latin/Black	Turn deep or bronze in sun	Cool or Deep Winter; Muted or Deep Autumn

MY SKINTONE IS _____

Remember, it's not one feature – the colour of your hair, eyes or skintone – that's important, but the picture the three create together that provides us with a guide to our best seasonal look.

HEALTH AND AGEING AFFECT COLOURING

As we age, our skintone, like our hair colour and eyes, softens and loses its intensity. After women pass through the menopause and experience a drop in oestrogen in their system the skin tone becomes 'less warm' in colouring than when they were younger. Melanin, the brown pigmentation in our skin which causes freckling and makes the skin look warm, may become more prominent later in life with the advent of 'age spots', but the basic overall skintone will be less warm. Hence later in life some women can begin wearing cooler tones.

We found from studying photographs of famous women, as well as our clients, that over a lifetime most of us will 'adjust' our seasonal colours and switch from one end of the spectrum to the other as we get older. A young auburn-haired, hazel-eyed Autumn looks most exciting in her deepest, spiciest colours. By her mid to late forties, when she begins to go grey, she might be better in more subtle colours. In other words a softer Autumn palette with more muted, warm tones would be more flattering as she ages.

When the Queen Mother was a young girl she had rich chestnut hair and sapphire eyes. She was a striking Clear Spring. As her hair began to turn grey she looked better and more harmonious if she wore the lighter Spring colours. Her ivory skintone was still beautifully warm but there was no longer the contrast between her hair and skin colour and she will have found the need to adjust her colours from bright jewel tones to warm pastels and elegant neutrals like ivory, stone, camel and warm greys.

In her seventies the Queen Mother went decidely 'cool'. Since then she glows in her blues, rosy pinks, sea greens and lemon yellows. No longer could she wear a coral tone lipstick, but she looks great in her favourite rose pink lipstick, which is so much more complimentary to the pink cast that her skin now has, and which is set off by her silver hair (no longer a warm grey) and her softer blue grey eyes. She's changed from being a Clear Spring to a Light Spring to now a Light Summer.

Switching seasons is not always necessary late in life, particularly if women continue to enhance their greying hair with rinses closer to its natural colour. But if you discovered your season some time ago and worry that some of the colours might now be a bit strong for you, read through the three options presented for your season (on pages 34–57) and see which one suits you best. One end of your seasonal spectrum might be more harmonious with your colouring today. If still unsure, start afresh in considering the possibilities for a woman with your current skintone, eye and hair colour.

Your diet, lifestyle and general health can all affect your colouring. Let's consider what you eat. Many women are keen to try new foods, diet regimes and supplements. Some dietary supplements, whether organic or artificial, and fanatical diets can build up harmful toxins in the body that can affect the colour of the skin as well as your health.

Your lifestyle can also create 'high' colour or 'low' colour. If hyperactive with stress regularly pumping your heart into overdrive you can look flushed and falsely 'warm' in skintone simply due to high blood pressure or a raised pulse rate. When you are calm and rested you might look very different, less pink, maybe more neutral in skin colour. Likewise when tired or lacklustre from a sedentary lifestyle with poor circulation you can appear paler in skintone than you might be if fit and active.

If you are unhealthy at present or treating a condition on prescription you might notice a change not only in your skin texture – the amount of dryness or oil secretions – but also in skin colour. Some prescriptions can make you look yellow or olive in tone when you are usually a natural beige or even pink.

So, if you are under any of the influences I've discussed put less of an emphasis on analysing the colour of your skintone and more on your overall key colouring characteristic as well as your eye colour and hair. Otherwise wait until you are fighting fit again and have regained your normal colouring before colour analysing yourself.

SHOPPING WITH YOUR COLOURS

Whatever your nationality and colouring, you will find that one of the 12 Seasonal Palettes is right for you. On pages 34–57 each Seasonal type is provided with an overall description of her colour range, along with 28 of her key colours and suggestions for business, evening and casual looks. Read this again every time you intend shopping for clothes, or, better still, take it with you. For a complete list of your seasonal colours, along with a Wardrobe Plan for Working Women, see pages 173–180. But please bear in mind that some colours are extremely difficult to reproduce exactly, even with super-efficient modern print technology – particularly when very many colours are shown together on a single page. They are, however, true enough to give you clear guidance when shopping on the range of colours that is best for you. You will also find advice on enhancing your seasonal colours through make-up on pages 34–57.

Don't get hung-up on matching colours exactly. Dyes, too, change every fashion season. Remember that as long as colours blend with your season and you can see them co-ordinating with other items in your wardrobe, you are on the right track; just avoid buying shades that are completely different from those recommended in your palette.

You will find that shopping is easier and you will no longer make mistakes or end up with impulse buys that don't go with anything else in your wardrobe – or you! The big plus is that you will save valuable time and money.

When you discover your season, you may realise that you have few of the recommended shades in your existing wardrobe. Don't worry; many of the 'unseasonal' colours that you already own can still be worn successfully, provided you team them with your right seasonal shades. Take black, for instance. Now this is a colour that seems to crop up in everyone's wardrobe. If black isn't in your season, all you have to do is wear the item with one of your favourite seasonal shades close to your face. Black trousers and skirts can be worn with a flattering blouse, jumper or jacket, while black dresses, tops, or big investment items like coats and jackets, can be worn with a scarf in your season's colours.

COLOURS FOR ALL SEASONS

Certain neutral colours, such as stone, pewter, soft white, medium navy and medium grey are readily available all year. Suits and other appropriate business clothes are often found in these neutrals, either singly or blended as in plaids, tweeds and prints; for example, a soft white, navy and pewter woven jacket.

These neutrals can be worn by all seasonal types, if the appropriate palette is brought into play. For example, in the summer, stone-coloured suits are on sale everywhere, with discount or designer labels. But a Warm Spring would wear her stone suit with an aqua blouse, while a Deep Winter could wear true red or black for greatest effect.

Medium navy and mid-tone grey are included with these neutrals because many women working in very conservative, male dominated sectors still need to play safe by wearing traditional business colours. Again, wear these neutrals with a complimentary shade from your seasonal palette. If you aren't restricted in your job or lifestyle, you can choose other neutrals and colours from your palette which you know to be more flattering.

Here are 10 colours that are complimentary to many skintones and usually available year round. They are also recommended for uniformed staff.

Soft white: As a blouse is always safer than pure white.

Stone: In a coat dress or suit, which can be offset with scarves in your season.

Warm pink: Always more flattering than cool, pastel, or fuchsia pink.

Medium turquoise: Not too bright, not too light. A 'user-friendly' shade.

Periwinkle: A blue violet we include in all CMB palettes.

Teal blue: A rich, deep green-blue – the CMB logo!

Emerald turquoise: Beautiful when mixed with navy, stone, or grey.

Medium purple: An elegant alternative to navy.

Medium navy: If required for work, choose mid-tone shades rather than inky or greyed versions. Team with something other than white if possible.

Soft charcoal, Medium grey: When in doubt both of these are better than very light, or near-black varieties.

TESTING YOUR SEASON: DEEP WOMEN

Our four models (opposite) all have rich, striking colouring with Diana and Harriet being the most delicate and Amrita and Ruth the strongest. Each will want to discern if she is more cool and complemented by the Winter colours or more warm and complemented by the Autumn colours.

Caucasian and Far East Asian women with Deep colouring should try make-up and fabric colours from the Deep palettes of Autumn and Winter to decide which colours are most natural and flattering to their skintone. Women with deeper skintones, like Amrita and Ruth, will need to see if the warmer shades of Autumn make their skin look muddy or jaundiced. More often, the Winter palette will work to clarify the skintone making it look brighter and healthier.

Try comparing the following colours near your face:

Autumn		Winter
Light Peach	vs.	Icy Pink
Ivory	vs.	Pure White
Marigold	vs.	Lemon Gold
Terracotta	vs.	Fuchsia

Now compare the following lip and cheek colours:

Autumn		Winter
Mahogany lipstick	vs.	Burgundy lipstick
Brick Red lipstick	vs.	Fuchsia lipstick
Cinnamon blush	vs.	Plum blush

Diana is a Deep Autumn and Harriet a Clear Winter while Amrita and Ruth are both Deep Winters.

THE TWELVE SEASONAL TYPES

Now we've got the essential preliminaries out of the way let's move on to the final decision making: which of the descriptions on pages 34–57 best fits you!

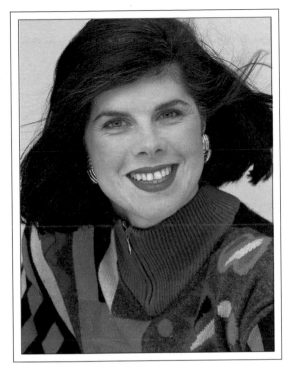

Harriet

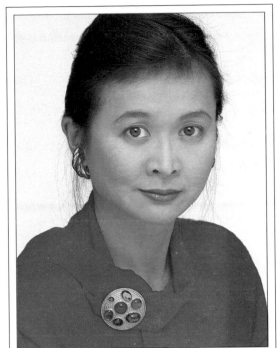

Diana

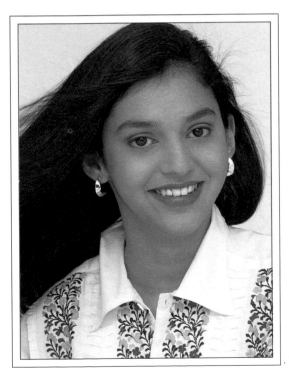

Amrita

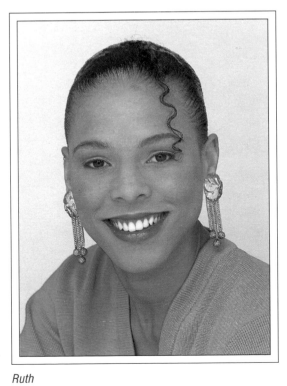

Ruth

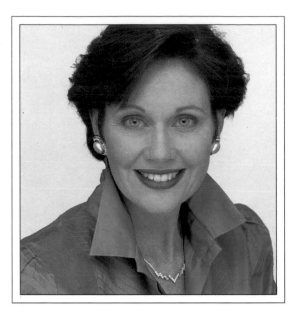

THE CLEAR SPRING

Overall look: Clear and contrasting

Hair: Medium to dark brown; salt 'n' pepper

Skintone: Very light and translucent. Porcelain, ivory or clear beige

Eyes: Jewel-like blue, blue-violet, green or bright hazel

IF the Clear Spring wears very dark, dusty colours, pale pastels or golden browns she looks boring, but in true blue, clear red or emerald green she looks wonderful. Bright, clear shades are her best.

The Clear Spring colouring is more warm than cool but still looks quite neutral when compared to the Warm Spring type. The key to the Clear Spring palette is that the colours are clear not muddy; see opposite. The colours are most exciting when worn in contrast; for example, ivory and red or charcoal and warm pastel pink.

Your most useful neutrals are the greys, ranging from light grey to charcoal. But black is also great for you, particularly if you have darker hair.

Blue-eyed Clear Springs won't look as good in the olive or the dark browns as the green- and hazel-eyed Clear Springs. Instead opt for your greys, blues and emerald turquoise colours.

Notice how true the blues, reds, greens and yellows are. These primary colours overwhelm other Seasons (except the Winters) but are dynamite on you.

Beware of beige, tan and muddy brown tones which take all the sparkle from your eyes and make your skin appear sallow.

Your alternative business look might be a versatile charcoal suit with a warm pink blouse. Black will be fine for evening, and hot turquoise is another good option; so are true red, emerald green and purple. For casual wear team up your reds, whites and blues.

Make-Up Tips

Foundation: Ivory, porcelain, clear beige **Lipstick**: Clear red, warm pink, strawberry **Blush**: Salmon, soft red **Eyeshadow** for blue or blue-violet eyes: *Highlighter* Champagne, soft pink, melon, pewter *Contour* Grey, navy, grape, teal **Eyeshadow** for clear green or hazel eyes: *Highlighter* Apricot, mint, lemon *Contour* Grey, spruce, deep brown, grape.

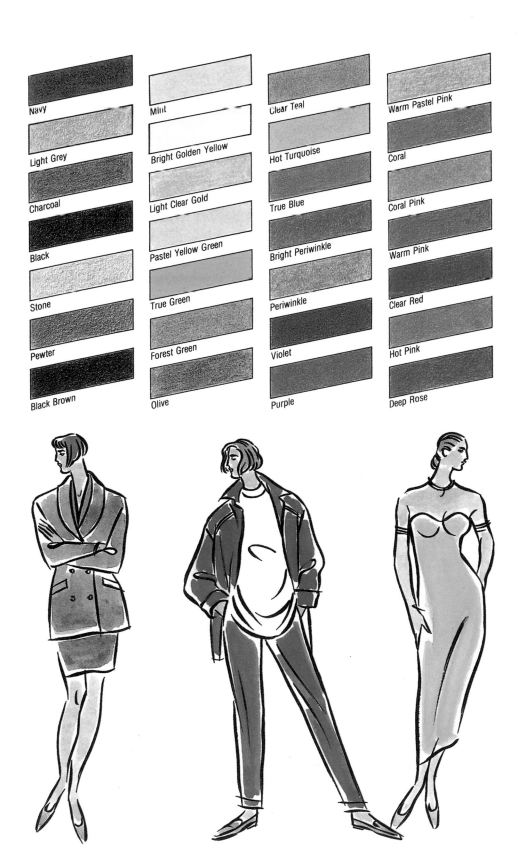

Navy

Light Grey

Charcoal

Black

Stone

Pewter

Black Brown

Mint

Bright Golden Yellow

Light Clear Gold

Pastel Yellow Green

True Green

Forest Green

Olive

Clear Teal

Hot Turquoise

True Blue

Bright Periwinkle

Periwinkle

Violet

Purple

Warm Pastel Pink

Coral

Coral Pink

Warm Pink

Clear Red

Hot Pink

Deep Rose

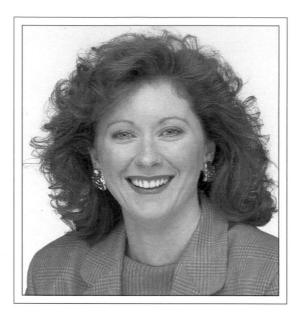

THE WARM SPRING

Overall look: Golden and clear

Hair: Golden or strawberry blonde, or red

Skintone: Ivory or porcelain; often with freckles

Eyes: Warm greens, teal blue, turquoise, or clear, light hazel

THE Warm Spring, like her Autumn counterpart, has an easy time understanding her colours – if they have a golden, rich glow they are probably good for you. Unlike the Warm Autumns, the Warm Spring has a more delicate, clear look so you'll take your colours only so deep. For example, the yellow greens are great for you, including moss, but forest green is too heavy.

Warm Springs must take particular care when choosing pinks, blues and reds, and must always select those with golden undertones. Coral pink will make you sparkle and look healthy, while blue-pinks such as fuchsia will completely drain your skintone and look harsh. This will also be true of your make-up (see below); any cool pinks will stand out and not look natural. Choose salmon, peach and apricot tones for best results.

See suggested colour combinations in the illustrations opposite for work, evening and play. Golden brown and aqua as a combination business suit will make you look both authoritative and interesting. Your alternative to black for the evening might be gold, which is stunning on you (but also consider emerald turquoise or deep periwinkle blue). Build your leisure wardrobe from the terracotta, golds and camels. You have endless possibilities, once you begin working with your beautiful Warm Spring palette.

Make-Up Tips

Foundation: Ivory, porcelain, warm beige   **Lipstick**: Warm pink, coral peach, spice   **Blush**: Salmon, spicy peach, light cinnamon   **Eyeshadow** for teal blue or turquoise eyes: *Highlighter* Apricot, lemon   *Contour* Teal, sea greens, grey, cocoa browns   **Eyeshadow** for green or hazel eyes: *Highlighter* Lemon, apricot, pea green   *Contour* Bronze/brown tones, plums, moss, sage, spruce.

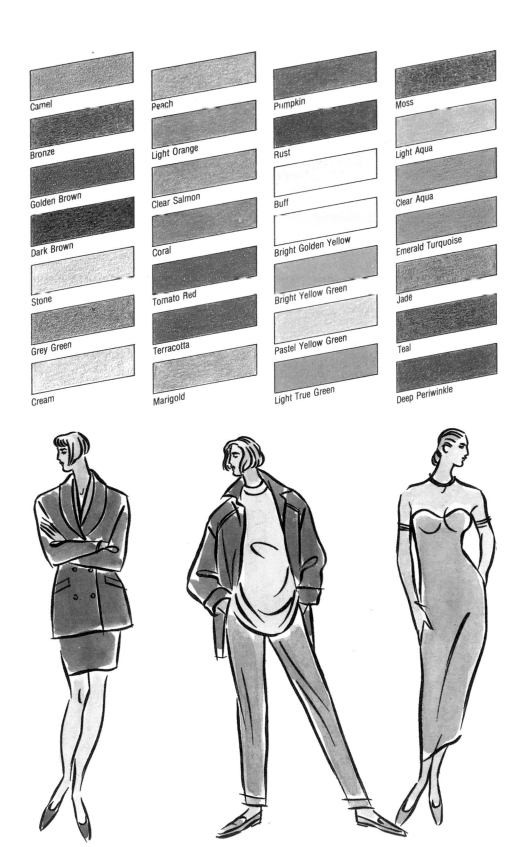

Camel

Bronze

Golden Brown

Dark Brown

Stone

Grey Green

Cream

Peach

Light Orange

Clear Salmon

Coral

Tomato Red

Terracotta

Marigold

Pumpkin

Rust

Buff

Bright Golden Yellow

Bright Yellow Green

Pastel Yellow Green

Light True Green

Moss

Light Aqua

Clear Aqua

Emerald Turquoise

Jade

Teal

Deep Periwinkle

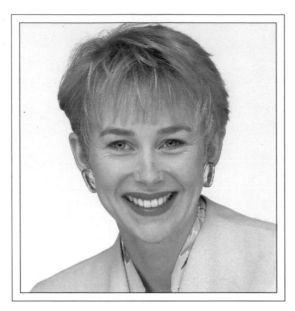

THE LIGHT SPRING

Overall look: Soft and delicate

Hair: Most often blonde or golden grey

Skintone: Light, ivory to soft beige, peachy tones. Very little contrast between hair and skin

Eyes: Blue, blue-green, aqua, light green

IF you are a Light Spring you should avoid dark and dusty colours, which would make you look pale, tired and even pathetic. Spring women who need to look strong, for example chairing a meeting, can do so by wearing mid-tone grey or light navy, not deeper shades.

If you are a Light Spring and you wear too much contrast, say a light blouse and dark jacket, or a dress with lots of bold colours against a white background, *you* 'disappear' because our eye is drawn to the colours you are wearing.

See your Light Spring palette opposite. Your neutrals can be worn singly or mixed with others in a print or weave. The ivory, camel and blue-greys are good investment shades that will work with any others in your palette. Your best pinks will be warm – see the peaches, corals and apricots – but also rose pink. Never go as far as fuchsia, which is too strong and would drain all the life from your skin.

Periwinkle blue toned with a light blue blouse is a smart, striking alternative to navy and white for work. Why wear black in the evening when you will sparkle in violet (also, warm pink and emerald turquoise will turn heads)? For leisure wear, team camel with clear bright red or khaki with salmon.

Make-Up Tips

Foundation: Ivory, porcelain   **Lipstick:** Peach, salmon, coral, clear red   **Blush:** Salmon, peach   **Eyeshadow** for blue eyes: *Highlighter* Champagne, melon, apricot, soft pink   *Contour* Soft grey, violet, teal blue, soft blues, cocoa   **Eyeshadow** for blue-green and aqua eyes: *Highlighter* Apricot, lemon, champagne   *Contour* Cocoa or honey brown, spruce or moss green, teal blue   **Eyeshadow** for green eyes: *Highlighter* Pale aqua, apricot, champagne   *Contour* Cocoa or honey brown, teal blue, violet, spruce.

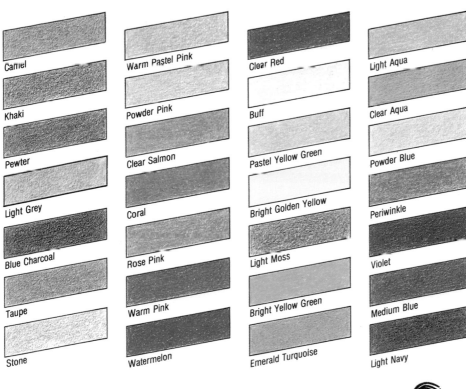

Camel

Khaki

Pewter

Light Grey

Blue Charcoal

Taupe

Stone

Warm Pastel Pink

Powder Pink

Clear Salmon

Coral

Rose Pink

Warm Pink

Watermelon

Clear Red

Buff

Pastel Yellow Green

Bright Golden Yellow

Light Moss

Bright Yellow Green

Emerald Turquoise

Light Aqua

Clear Aqua

Powder Blue

Periwinkle

Violet

Medium Blue

Light Navy

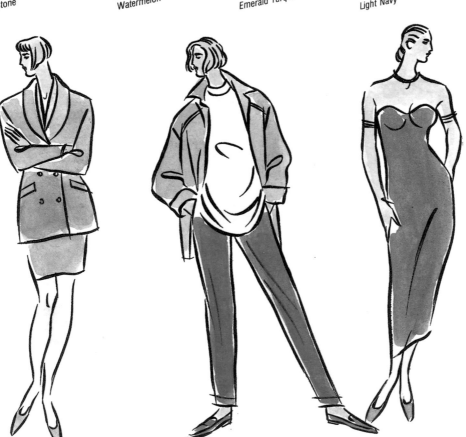

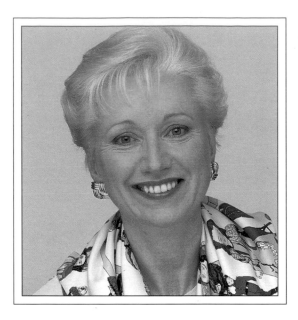

THE LIGHT SUMMER

Overall look: Soft and delicate

Hair: Ash blonde, grey blonde, cool grey

Skintone: Ivory, soft or cool beige

Eyes: Soft blue, blue-grey, grey

THE Light Summer can look elegant or older than her years, depending on the colours she wears. Her elegance comes from dressing in the colours of a July garden – like the sweet peas, pinks, lavenders, periwinkles and dusty roses. If this is you, aim to avoid very dark colours which will make you look much older, or bright colours that will simply look inexpensive on you.

While you may be able to wear stronger colours early in life, the older Light Summer knows that her grey or ash hair are best complemented by soft blue greys, light pink to deep rose tones, pink browns and blue-greens.

See the Light Summer palette opposite. Notice how blended and harmonious the colours appear. There's not much contrast in the palette, so your most interesting use of colour will result when you blend shades monochromatically; for example, deep periwinkle, lavender and dusty rose.

The wide choice of aquas and blue-greens give you fresh alternatives to blues which you, no doubt, have in plenty in your wardrobe already.

Your reds range from a clear watermelon to the rich blue-reds, but burgundy is too strong for your light colouring.

Grey-blue is a great neutral for a work suit. Try wearing it with lavender (as shown), or pastel pinks.

Black is definitely not for you – it drains you of all life and colour. Rose or soft teal will be winning alternatives for evening.

For leisure hours, medium blues and navies can be livened up by mixing them with clear aqua (as shown) or emerald turquoise.

Make-Up Tips

Foundation: Ivory, rose beige, cool beige   **Lipstick**: Dusty rose, soft plum, rose pink   **Blush**: Soft rose   **Eyeshadow** for soft blues, blue-grey or grey eyes: *Highlighter* Soft pink, lemon, pewter, champagne   *Contour* Grey, blue-grey, soft teal, slate, plum, cocoa.

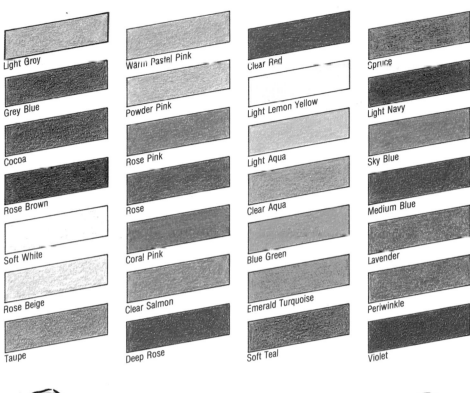

Light Grey

Grey Blue

Cocoa

Rose Brown

Soft White

Rose Beige

Taupe

Warm Pastel Pink

Powder Pink

Rose Pink

Rose

Coral Pink

Clear Salmon

Deep Rose

Clear Red

Light Lemon Yellow

Light Aqua

Clear Aqua

Blue Green

Emerald Turquoise

Soft Teal

Spruce

Light Navy

Sky Blue

Medium Blue

Lavender

Periwinkle

Violet

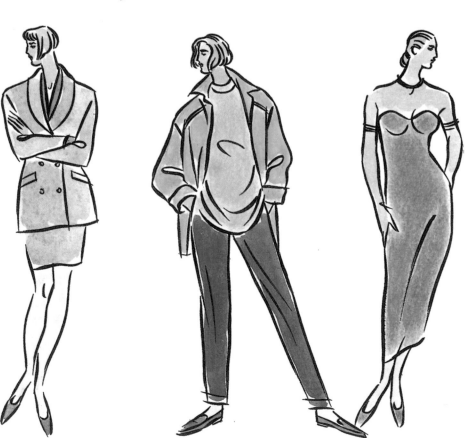

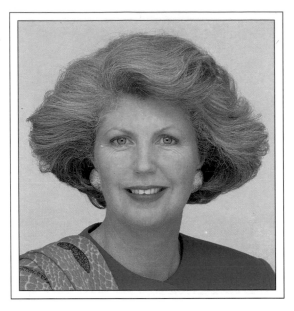

THE COOL SUMMER

Overall look: Cool and soft

Hair: Ash brown, deep ash blonde or grey

Skintone: Soft pink, beige, rose beige

Eyes: Grey, grey-blue or blue-green

THE Cool Summer probably already has a wardrobe full of blue. But the Cool Summer who only wears pastel, insipid shades can look unexciting. If this is you, your best blues range from blue greys through to rich royal and deep navy.

A key point to remember is to steer clear of warm tones – thus golden browns, orange reds and yellow greens are all disappointing on you. The pink undertones to your skin and your grey, grey-blue or green eyes are best complemented by the greys. Taupe, a grey-beige and cocoa, rose beige and rose browns are all fine, due to their pink, cool undertones.

All Summers, including the Cool type, look best in blended shades. Even though you have navy, burgundy, purple and charcoal grey included in your palette, soften the effect of these by teaming them not with white, but rather a pastel version of the colour itself.

See the Cool Summer palette opposite. These colours are just representative of a huge range of possibilities, provided the shade will blend with your Cool Summer colours. Navy, as you probably know, will be a useful staple for work. Try it with rose for a softer look.

Black is too heavy for the Cool Summer. For evening try soft teal (soft fuchsia, plum and blue-red are also good choices). Your leisurewear might be in medium grey and emerald turquoise but your navies and blue-greys are also a possibility.

Make-Up Tips

Foundation: Ivory, rose beige, cool beige   **Lipstick**: Raspberry, plum rose, red geranium, soft mauve, fuchsia   **Blush**: Rose, soft mauve, soft fuchsia
Eyeshadow for grey-blue eyes: *Highlighter* Soft pink, champagne, pearl grey *Contour* Steel grey, navy, plum   **Eyeshadow** for blue-green eyes: *Highlighter* Apricot, lemon, mint, champagne *Contour* Grey, plum, spruce.

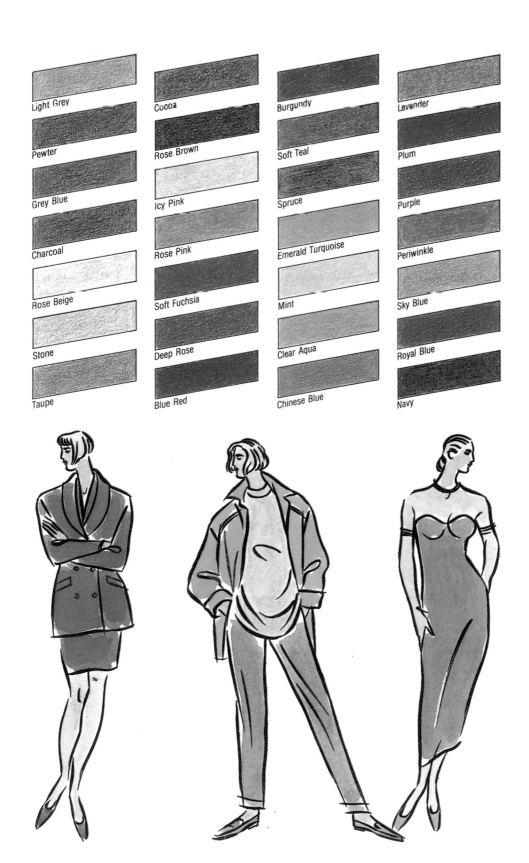

Light Grey

Pewter

Grey Blue

Charcoal

Rose Beige

Stone

Taupe

Cocoa

Rose Brown

Icy Pink

Rose Pink

Soft Fuchsia

Deep Rose

Blue Red

Burgundy

Soft Teal

Spruce

Emerald Turquoise

Mint

Clear Aqua

Chinese Blue

Lavender

Plum

Purple

Periwinkle

Sky Blue

Royal Blue

Navy

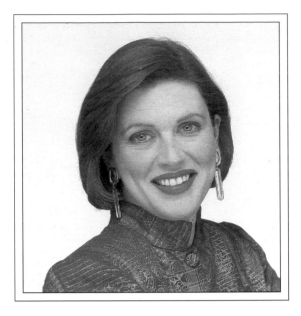

THE SOFT SUMMER

Overall look: Muted and dusty

Hair: Ash blonde, medium brown, mousy grey

Skintone: Ivory, beige

Eyes: Soft teal, grey-green, blue-grey, soft hazel

THE Soft Summer has a natural elegance to her colouring that is very special, but often these women despair at looking 'mousy' or 'uninteresting'. It is true that if the Soft Summer wears very strong or bright colours she is not only overpowered by them but can, indeed, look mousy. However, when she wears blended colours her hair and skin take on a new vitality. If you are a Soft Summer there is no need to resort to chemical highlights in your hair (unless you want them) because your beautiful palette of rich, blended tones will always make you look healthy and interesting.

See the Soft Summer palette opposite. No colour jumps out at you. The colour choice ranges from light but substantive pastels like mint, blue-green, rose beige and soft white to rich burgundy, amethyst and teal. Nothing neon or electric for the elegant Soft Summer.

For work, lovely jade when combined with a rich rose creates an elegant, professional presence.

You realise that black is unsuccessful for you unless worn away from the face, say, in skirts or trousers. So be different, be yourself, and choose alternative colours that will make you look wonderful after dark. We've suggested pewter in our illustration but spruce or forest green are also well worth considering.

For relaxing, raspberry is an easy choice for basics, and just waiting to be combined with mauve, medium blue or cocoa. But watermelon red will always create a vibrant alternative for the Soft Summer.

Make-Up Tips

Foundation: Ivory, beige **Lipstick**: Tan pink, dusty rose, plum rose **Blush**: Pinky brown, soft plum, rose **Eyeshadow** for soft teal or blue-grey eyes: *Highlighter* Soft pink, mint, lemon, champagne *Contour* Teal, smoky grey, plum, navy **Eyeshadow** for grey-green or soft hazel eyes: *Highlighter* Lemon, opal, apricot *Contour* Plum, smoky grey, cocoa, jade.

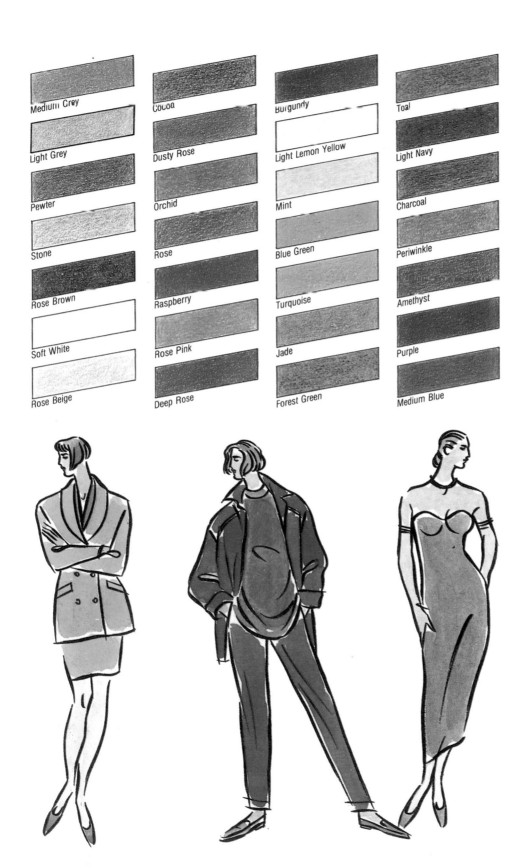

Medium Grey

Light Grey

Pewter

Stone

Rose Brown

Soft White

Rose Beige

Cocoa

Dusty Rose

Orchid

Rose

Raspberry

Rose Pink

Deep Rose

Burgundy

Light Lemon Yellow

Mint

Blue Green

Turquoise

Jade

Forest Green

Toal

Light Navy

Charcoal

Periwinkle

Amethyst

Purple

Medium Blue

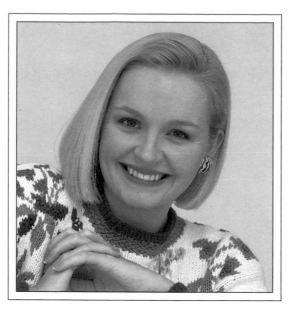

THE SOFT AUTUMN

Overall look: Rich and muted

Hair: Medium brown, golden blonde, mousy brown/ blonde

Skintone: Beige

Eyes: Hazel, topaz, brown, grey-green

THE Soft Autumn has strength about her colouring that often eludes her and others. If she dresses in very dark cool colours, navy for example, she looks pale and uninteresting. Black is particularly unkind to the Soft Autumn and when worn elicits comments like 'are you feeling all right?'.

If you are a Soft Autumn then to look healthy and vibrant choose rich elegant shades. Unlike the Warm Autumn you can't wear the oranges and mustards but most Soft Autumns instinctively turn away from these shades anyway.

See the Soft Autumn palette opposite. Your pinks range from soft peaches and salmons to deep rose – a soft blend of warm and cool tones because your colouring is quite neutral. Any of these pinks are terrific worn alone or with your best useful basics, say olive, coffee or stone.

Dark navies and greys, the good old standby business colours, are *not* good for you. But if you need to wear them, enhance the effect with blouses in favourite colours from your palette. Otherwise substitute pewter for grey, which is more flattering to your colouring. And doesn't it look wonderful with salmon?

For evening, your best choice is purple. Imagine it in a rich satin, wool crêpe or raw silk.

For relaxing, olive green is the most versatile neutral (also great for suits). Mahogany and bronze with a dash of buttermilk or bittersweet is also a timeless combination that can be worn all year round.

Make-Up Tips
Foundation: Ivory, beige   **Lipstick**: Spiced peach, mahogany, terracotta, brick red, tan pink   **Blush**: Cinnamon, salmon, spiced peach   **Eyeshadow** for hazel, topaz, brown, or grey-green eyes: *Highlighter* Apricot, lemon, champagne   *Contour* Bronze, moss, olive, purple, brown, warm grey.

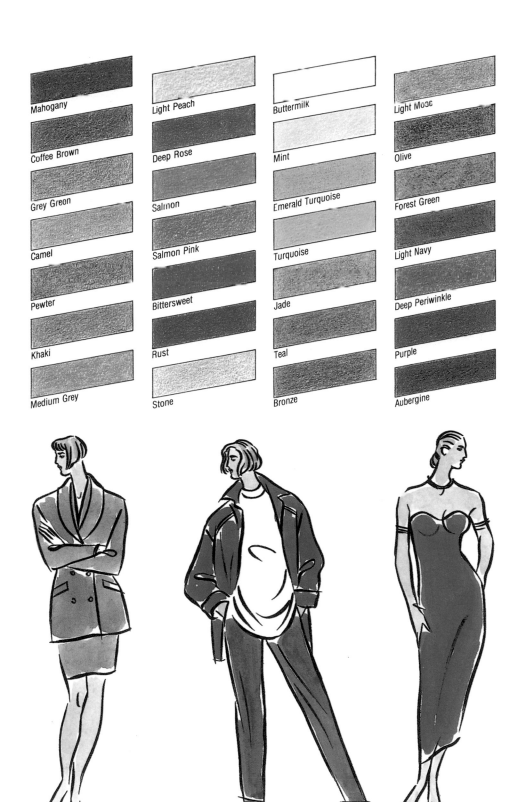

Mahogany

Coffee Brown

Grey Green

Camel

Pewter

Khaki

Medium Grey

Light Peach

Deep Rose

Salmon

Salmon Pink

Bittersweet

Rust

Stone

Buttermilk

Mint

Emerald Turquoise

Turquoise

Jade

Teal

Bronze

Light Mose

Olive

Forest Green

Light Navy

Deep Periwinkle

Purple

Aubergine

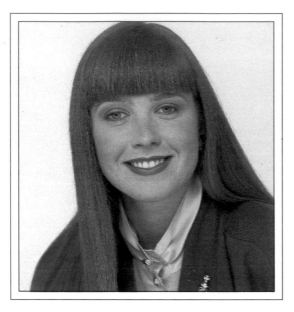

THE WARM AUTUMN

Overall Look: Golden and rich

Hair: Auburn, red, golden blonde

Skintone: Warm beige, ivory often with freckles

Eyes: Topaz, hazel, warm green, teal blue

IF any seasonal type had an easy time shopping it is the Warm Autumn; designers love to work in your rich, spicy colours. Imagine walking through a golden wood on a sunny autumnal day when the leaves all start to change colour and you'll have the feel of this glorious palette.

See the range of colours in the Warm Autumn palette opposite. Rich coffee, camel and golden brown will be the staples of your wardrobe. But don't be unimaginative when using these colours; team them up with bittersweet red, emerald turquoise or purple.

Notice your reds have yellow or orange undertones. Burgundy reds or blue-pinks are not for you because they would drain all the colour from your face. It is the warm reds that enhance your natural golden glow and make those freckles (if you have them) an asset not a liability.

Let's consider how you can use the Warm Autumn shades to dress for success. Although grey and navy are in your palette (see page 175) if you don't need to wear these traditional colours, don't. A better combination would be bronze and bittersweet red.

What about evening wear? Imagine elegant pewter in a rich silk jersey – or periwinkle or teal are two other terrific bets to outshine everyone else in their 'safe' little black numbers.

At home, coffees and camels will be good wardrobe basics for trousers, skirts, sweaters, etcetera. But why not exploit your beautiful natural colouring with mustard, terracotta and aubergine?

Make-Up Tips

Foundation: Ivory, warm beige   **Lipstick**: Terracotta, cinnamon, brick red   **Blush**: Terracotta, salmon, spice   **Eyeshadow** for topaz, hazel or warm green eyes: *Highlighter* Apricot, light gold, pea green, champagne   *Contour* Bronze, brown, medium purple, spruce, moss.

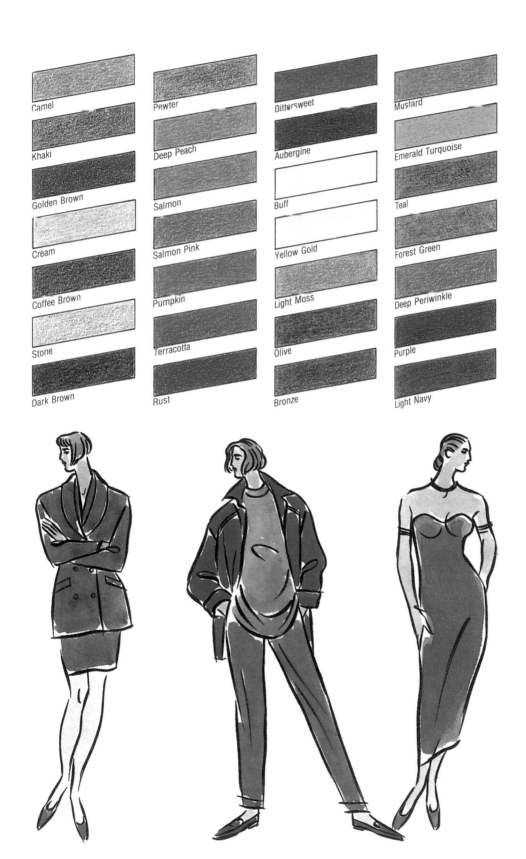

Camel

Khaki

Golden Brown

Cream

Coffee Brown

Stone

Dark Brown

Pewter

Deep Peach

Salmon

Salmon Pink

Pumpkin

Terracotta

Rust

Bittersweet

Aubergine

Buff

Yellow Gold

Light Moss

Olive

Bronze

Mustard

Emerald Turquoise

Teal

Forest Green

Deep Periwinkle

Purple

Light Navy

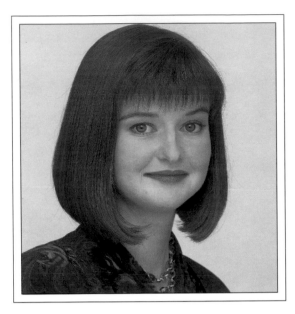

THE DEEP AUTUMN

Overall look: Vivid and warm

Hair: Deep brown, chestnut, auburn

Skintone: Honey brown, bronze, black, golden olive, warm beige, ivory

Eyes: Rich olive or hazel, golden brown, black-brown

THE Deep Autumn is most exciting in vivid striking colours that are mostly warm in undertone. Your strong colouring demands deep shades worn with bright or light ones for contrast.

See the Deep Autumn palette opposite. Colours that would certainly be too strong for a Spring or Summer make the Deep Autumn look dynamic. As for the Soft Autumn, olive is a great neutral but the Deep Autumn woman will wear it boldly, with hot turquoise or terracotta.

The strength of this Deep Autumn palette requires you to take particular care with your make-up. Recommended shades are listed below. But remember that when wearing bold colours you need to balance them in your make-up; no dashing out bare-faced. In tomato or true red you are no less than wonderful, but your make-up must complete the effect with matching lipstick.

For business, an olive suit is very versatile – in gaberdine for winter time or in linen for summer time. But your tomato red would create a stunning effect if co-ordinated with an olive blouse. Both of these colours offer unlimited possibilities with the rest of your palette.

Black is great on you but when you are feeling more adventurous, try dark brown in a rich velvet. Black and Asian women might prefer Chinese blue.

An excellent idea is to try rust, lime or terracotta with black or black-brown basics to make your weekend and casual gear easy to co-ordinate.

Make-Up Tips
Foundation: Ivory, warm beige, bronze   **Lipstick**: Terracotta, true red, cinnamon   **Blush**: Cinnamon, red, terracotta   **Eyeshadow** for olive or hazel eyes: *Highlighter* Apricot, pea green, lemon, melon   *Contour* Bronze, olive, sage, purple, grey, brown   **Eyeshadow** for golden brown or black-brown eyes: *Highlighter* Apricot, lemon, pea green   *Contour* Grey, spruce, olive, purple.

Pewter

Black Brown

Stone

Black

Cream

Camel

Light Peach

Deep Peach

Salmon Pink

Tomato Red

Mahogany

True Red

Terracotta

Rust

Aubergine

Yellow Gold

Mustard

Moss

Olive

Lime

Bronze

Emerald Green

Hot Turquoise

Chinese Blue

Pine

Navy

Teal

Purple

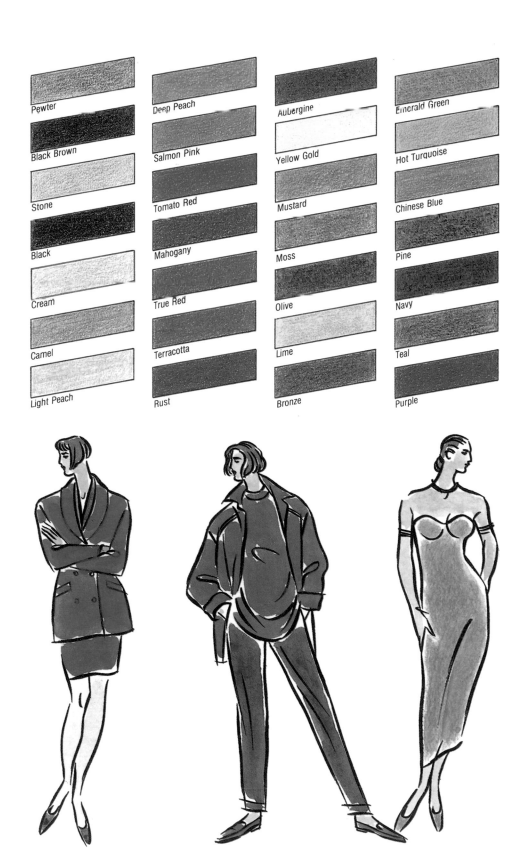

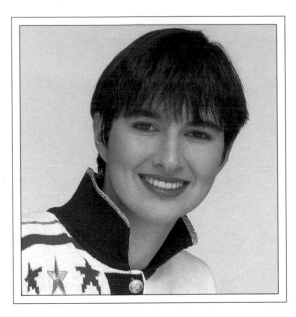

THE DEEP WINTER

Overall look: Deep and cool

Hair: Dark brown, black, deepest auburn

Skintone: Black, cool brown, olive, cool beige

Eyes: Deep brown, hazel, olive

THE Deep Winter can successfully wear combinations of dark colours which would make other seasonal types pale into insignificance. Your brown hair could never be called mousy – it's the strongest chestnut, auburn or, as with dark skins, it may even have a blue cast. Your eyes are also strong. Your skintone could not be called delicate either; it, too, has strength – cool beige, olive or brown.

The only way to complement such colouring is to choose vibrant primaries, deep neutrals and rich versatile shades that can be blended according to your mood and personality.

For business, Deep Winters can make a striking impact in black (which figures prominently in your wardrobe), charcoal and navies. Charcoal with turquoise is a winning combination. You can be sure black will be stunning on you for evening wear but why not try true red for your next purchase – in satin, velvet or silk jersey? Dark-skinned Deep Winters are advised not to wear black or black-brown in large amounts, particularly near the face. You need to choose from the primary tones and contrasting shades to help brighten your striking features, rather than very dark tones that blend too closely with your own colouring.

For leisurewear, pine green and hot pink are winners on Deep Winters. But consider a lemon yellow jogging suit, or a true red sweater and charcoal jeans as exciting alternatives.

Make-Up Tips
Foundation: Warm beige, bronze, beige   **Lipstick**: True red, burgundy, plum, mahogany   **Blush**: Red, bronze, plum   **Eyeshadow** for deep brown, hazel, or olive eyes: *Highlighter* Apricot, lemon, champagne, mint   *Contour* Black-brown, grey, purple, spruce, olive, aubergine.

Black

Charcoal

Black Brown

Pewter

Brown Burgundy

Pure White

Stone

Icy Grey

Medium Grey

Hot Pink

True Red

Tomato Red

Burgundy

Rust

Blue Red

Mint

Lemon Yellow

Turquoise

Emerald Green

Olive

Pine

Emerald Turquoise

Clear Teal

Bright Periwinkle

Chinese Blue

Purple

True Blue

Navy

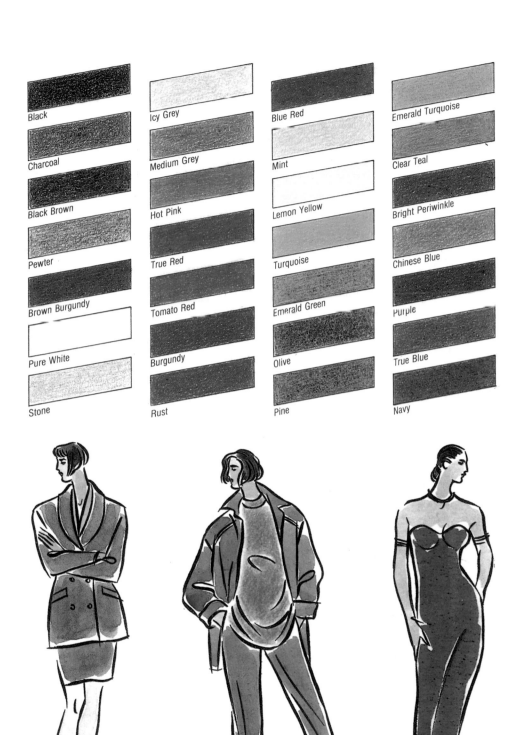

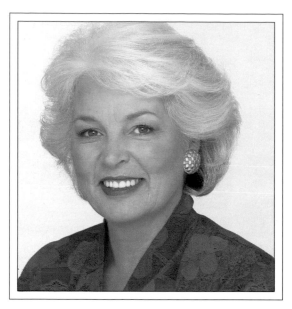

THE COOL WINTER

Overall look: Clear and cool

Hair: Silver grey, salt 'n' pepper, black-grey

Skintone: Ivory, clear olive, cool beige

Eyes: Deep brown, grey-brown

IF you are a Cool Winter you were probably a Deep Winter earlier in life but with the grey now coming through in your hair, and with your eyes and skintone softening, you are better avoiding the warmer tones that are vital to the Deep Winter, such as tomato red, olive and rust. Instead you should now go for the cool, softer colours from the Cool Winter palette such as plum, raspberry, fuchsia and blue-red.

See the harmony in the Cool Winter palette. Unlike other palettes that do blend some cool and warm colours, you can see that these colours all have the same cool undertone. Since your grey hair is a major feature, you will be best advised to use charcoal or true grey as your neutrals. Golden browns or beiges would make your hair look dull and lifeless, when in fact it is a wonderful asset.

For business, all Winters have an easier time than other seasonal types. Greys and navies look wonderful on Winters and are available throughout the year. But, as a Cool Winter you need to appreciate that when you wear traditional business combinations, the dark suit and light blouse (perhaps in navy and white), you can look older and rather severe. A softer suit teamed with a darker blouse – for example raspberry with taupe – gives good contrast and projects authority without making you unapproachable. Other choices for suits will be weaves of soft white, navy and grey. Plum or blue-red are also good.

For evening, black might be too severe. Why not opt for royal blue, in a silk chiffon crêpe jersey or taffeta? For relaxing, bright periwinkle blue and charcoal or icy grey would make a sensational combination.

Make-Up Tips

Foundation: Ivory, cool beige   **Lipstick:** Raspberry, plum rose, strawberry, soft fuchsia   **Blush:** Deep rose, plum, soft fuchsia   **Eyeshadow** for deep or grey-brown eyes: *Highlighter* Soft pink, icy grey, lemon, champagne *Contour* Slate, plum, grey, aubergine.

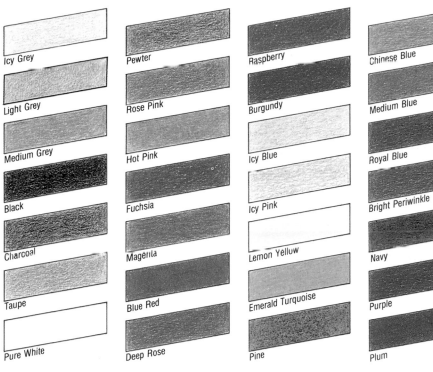

Icy Grey

Light Grey

Medium Grey

Black

Charcoal

Taupe

Pure White

Pewter

Rose Pink

Hot Pink

Fuchsia

Magenta

Blue Red

Deep Rose

Raspberry

Burgundy

Icy Blue

Icy Pink

Lemon Yellow

Emerald Turquoise

Pine

Chinese Blue

Medium Blue

Royal Blue

Bright Periwinkle

Navy

Purple

Plum

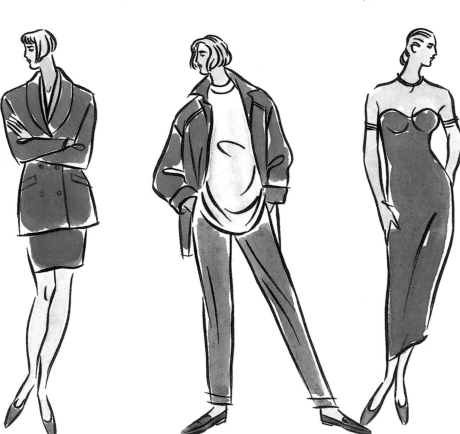

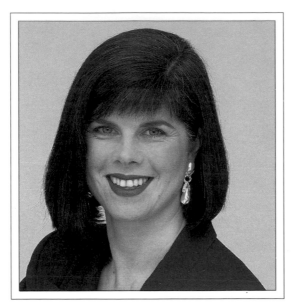

THE CLEAR WINTER

Overall look: Clear and contrasting

Hair: Black, dark brown, salt 'n' pepper, silver

Skintone: Porcelain, ivory, beige, clear olive

Eyes: Deep or violet blue, clear hazel

THE Clear Winter is similar to the Clear Spring but, overall has greater strength of colouring. Also, she often has striking, deep eyebrows to frame her remarkable jewel-like eyes and looks more interesting in the vibrant Winter colours and make-up tones than in the lighter Spring palette. Is this you?

The scope of the Clear Winter palette, opposite, is striking, too. Black and charcoal will all be terrific on you but look best if offset with lighter shades. Dark brown is an exciting neutral, but looks better on hazel- not blue-eyed Clear Winters. The Clear Winter looks stunning when contrasting light bright colours with dark ones. The very pale 'icy colours' are not mere pastels but the very palest shades of blue, pink, violet, yellow and grey. But don't wear these colours on their own – team them with richer shades, such as icy violet with purple; icy pink with charcoal grey; icy blue with pine green.

The Clear Winter has an easy time with business colours. Navies and greys are great on you. A royal blue suit offset with a fine knit black jersey will command everyone's attention. Look for weaves with taupe, grey and navy blended together, which can be co-ordinated with the same plain colours.

In the evening, black will be fine. For a change, however, emerald turquoise will help you sparkle. Also try hot pink, true blue or violet.

When you are relaxing, don't retreat into sludgy shades but keep your bright contrast. Try mixing clear teal and hot pink for fun.

Make-Up Tips

Foundation: Ivory, cool beige, porcelain **Lipstick**: Pinks from hot pink to strawberry, true reds, clear not dark plum **Blush**: Red, plum, hot pink **Eyeshadow** for deep- to violet-blue eyes: *Highlighter* Pink, icy violet, lemon, champagne *Contour* Slate, plum, grey **Eyeshadow** for clear hazel eyes: *Highlighter* Apricot, lemon, champagne, mint *Contour* Spruce, plum, grey, brown.

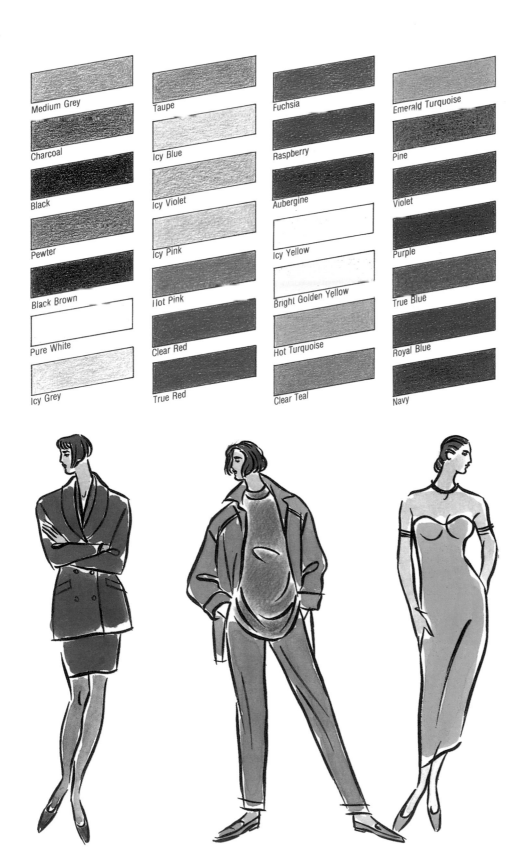

Medium Grey

Charcoal

Black

Pewter

Black Brown

Pure White

Icy Grey

Taupe

Icy Blue

Icy Violet

Icy Pink

Hot Pink

Clear Red

True Red

Fuchsia

Raspberry

Aubergine

Icy Yellow

Bright Golden Yellow

Hot Turquoise

Clear Teal

Emerald Turquoise

Pine

Violet

Purple

True Blue

Royal Blue

Navy

chapter four

Your colour vitamins

DID you know that certain colours you wear can actually affect you and others psychologically and physically, as well as aesthetically? In fact, wearing specific colours can help to elicit the right reaction from people in different situations. When you're very tired, for example, but still need to perform and perhaps have a presentation to deliver, if you wear a red suit you will not only give yourself an artificial boost of energy but will also command your audience's attention. And red isn't the only colour with subtle powers.

Such colours can be so effective that I like to refer to them as colour vitamins. There are eleven key colour vitamins – red, pink, blue, brown, yellow, green, orange, violet, grey, black and white. In the following pages you will find advice on how to use each of these colours for the best effect. But note that there are situations when you should actually *avoid* wearing certain colours – so I give these too.

COLOUR VITAMIN **|RED**

Includes: True, warm, burnished, bright and cool variations. Not shades that are too light (such as pink), mixed (as in fuchsia), or too dark (such as burgundy).

Psychological Power of Red
Positive attributes: Up-beat, confident, assertive, exciting.
Negative attributes: Aggressive, domineering, bossy, threatening.

Wearing Red for Emotional and Physical Impact
- Choose for occasions when you want to be recognised, or to catch someone's eye.

- Can give you an artificial boost of energy when tired.

- A great asset in attracting the opposite sex, but beware that it can overwhelm and backfire.

- To project authority without being threatening, wear red as an accent or in moderation; for example, as a blouse teamed with a neutral grey or taupe suit.

Avoid Wearing Red When
- Overtired or overstressed as it can exacerbate internal and external tension.

- Not prepared to be called upon to defend your position, as you would be signalling that you are.

- Meeting potential in-laws, you'll scare them.

- Being interviewed for a job you want; you'll give the impression that you're only concerned about yourself and not a team player.

- Chairing a staff meeting when you want your colleagues to generate the ideas. They won't dare make suggestions for fear of disagreeing with you.

- On television as it has a tendency to 'bleed' or go fuzzy at the edges, which looks very strange. Only the most elaborate, high-tech sets can handle red-suited guests.

COLOUR VITAMIN |PINK

Includes: The cotton-candy hues, both cool and warm, the mid-tone salmons, corals and raspberry pinks.

Psychological Power of Pink
Positive Attributes: Feminine, gentle, accessible, non-threatening.
Negative Attributes: Pathetic, unimportant, safe, under-confident.

Wearing Pink for Emotional and Physical Impact
- To soften an austere business look as a blouse or scarf to complement a neutral suit.

- For afternoon tea, christenings, and garden parties to look elegant.

- As grandmother of the bride.

- As a petitioner in Divorce Court. You'll win the sympathy of everyone including your husband's lawyer.

Avoid Wearing Pink When

● Discussing a promotion with your boss. Pink is not management material.

● At a client dinner, or keep in moderation, such as lipstick only.

● You are in the role of seducer (unless it's a warm, deep pink).

COLOUR VITAMIN |BLUE

Includes: True, royal, navy, clear and medium blues; however, not pale pastel versions or aquas.

Psychological Power of Blue
Positive Attributes: Peaceful, trustworthy, constant, orderly
Negative Attributes: 'Holier than Thou', tiresome, predictable, conservative

Wearing Blue for Emotional and Physical Impact

● The deepest blues project the most authority – just think of the uniform worn by police. If you want to look like the woman in charge, a navy or deep blue suit usually does the trick.

● Mid-tone blues produce the right effect on potential mothers-in-law, inspiring confidence that you'll take care of her little boy.

● On television, the mid-tone blues are the most 'media-friendly'.

When to Avoid Wearing Blue

● Making a creative pitch in PR, advertising, design or marketing. Blue and creativity are not generally felt to be synonymous.

● At a conference of bankers, lawyers, accountants or insurance salesmen, unless your objective is not to stand out.

● For a school reunion when you want to project success and confidence.

COLOUR VITAMIN |BROWN

Includes: Golden, chocolate, charcoal, cocoa and rose browns.

Psychological Power of Brown
Positive Attributes: Earthy, homely, gregarious.
Negative Attributes: Safe, boring, unsophisticated.

Wearing Brown for Emotional and Physical Impact
- To get people to open-up and communicate more freely, wear your season's best brown – the least threatening colour to others; investigative journalists take note!

- As an alternative to grey or navy in business (particularly if you are a Warm Spring or Warm Autumn). 'No man of renown wears brown,' perhaps, but successful women can easily and effectively use brown for business. We're only beginning to set standards for ourselves. Men have centuries of tradition to chip away at.

- When entertaining the in-laws. Brown creates the impression of being a successful Earth Mother to husband and kiddies even if you aren't.

When to Avoid Wearing Brown
- If positioning for a mangement buy-out of your company as you won't look like you're prepared for the risks ahead.

- When meeting friends with 'personal problems' as they'll pour their hearts out.

- For an elegant evening occasion, unless it's the most fabulous brown velvet, satin or lace.

- When hoping to attract the attention of someone who attracts *you* as it simply won't help your prospects.

- Among executive wives, you'll disappear into the woodwork.

COLOUR VITAMIN **YELLOW**

Includes: Sunny, bright and banana versions, through to gold, but not pastel shades like lemon.

Psychological Power of Yellow
Positive Attributes: Cheerful, hopeful, active, uninhibited.
Negative Attributes: Impulsive, tiresome, whirlwind, volatile.

Wearing Yellow for Emotional and Physical Impact
- To cheer yourself up, particularly on a dreary day.

- When in a fun mood and free to act irresponsibly.

- If working with children – it's the colour children prefer more than any other.

- On your birthday, especially if celebrating alone.

- Best as a jacket, if you want to be recognised in a crowd.

When to Avoid Wearing Yellow

- Negotiating the terms of a divorce settlement; yellow has frivolous connotations so wear your brown or pink vitamins instead.

- Advising a son or daughter about the facts of life – they won't take you seriously.

- In a business meeting if you don't have anything to contribute to the discussion; yellow makes you stand out.

- When asking your bank manager for an overdraft – you'll look a poor risk.

- If you live in a sunny climate; all yellows turn electric in bright light.

COLOUR VITAMIN **GREEN**

Includes: Olive, moss, forest, spruce, pine and true greens (not too yellow or too blue).

Psychological Power of Green
Positive Attributes: Self-reliant, tenacious, nurturing, dependable.
Negative Attributes: Boring, stubborn, risk averse, predictable.

Wearing Green for Emotional and Physical Impact

- When over-stressed and overtired, green produces restorative results.

- After days of more flamboyant use of colour, green helps bring you 'down-to-earth' creating a more balanced, level-headed feeling.

- Deep tones, such as forest, olive or pine green, are viable alternatives to navy for business.

- At a Friends of the Earth Bean Feast.

When to Avoid Wearing Green

- When fund raising. Research has proven that (even for Friends of the Earth) people will either bolt past you or give you lame excuses for not donating.

- As a rallying colour for a political movement (sorry, Green Party). It doesn't project new ideas but rather dated, backward thinking.

- To turn heads in the evening, unless it's emerald in silk or satin.

- As an entrepreneur with cap in hand to the bank manager or venture capitalist; you won't convince them that you have the vision or drive to succeed.

COLOUR VITAMIN | ORANGE

Includes: True orange, pumpkin, tangerine, bright peach.

Psychological Power of Orange

Postive Attributes: Vitality, fun, enthusiasm, sociability, uninhibited.
Negative Attributes: Superficial, common, faddist, giddy.

Wearing Orange for Emotional and Physical Impact

- Wear only if you are a Warm Spring or Autumn, and then in measured doses.

- If you want to be seen in the dark; try a neon orange jogging suit, or an orange jacket if you are riding a bike.

- If you want an energising colour and you have an 'invisible' job, such as a lab. technician or DJ.

When to Avoid Wearing Orange

- For business of any kind; orange is the least professional colour.

- Afternoon tea, in any setting; it's too elegant an occasion for orange!

- When dieting as you are more prone to act impulsively in orange and less likely to maintain self-control (hence, MacDonald's interior decorating).

- When you want to look elegant, as orange is a 'declassifier' and looks cheap on some seasonal types.

COLOUR VITAMIN | VIOLET

Includes: Mixtures of red and blue from periwinkle blue, clear or medium violet to purple, plum and indigo.

Psychological Power of Violet

Positive Attributes: Imaginative, sensitive, intuitive, unusual, unselfish.
Negative Attributes: Weird, impractical, immature, superior.

Wearing Violet for Emotional and Physical Impact

- In business situations where you need to project confidence and individuality. Mid-tone to deep purples are both appropriate and professional in business (and a welcome alternative to the navies and greys in traditional sectors).

- A winner on television; provided it is not too dark.

- Good when suggesting a new approach to an old problem. On any occasion requiring diplomacy.

- As an alternative to black for evening elegance, charm and seduction.

When to Avoid Wearing Violet

- Whenever a low-key yet reassuring profile is most appropriate.

- When interviewing for a limited place on an MBA programme, purple is too individualistic, non-conformist; who needs a troublesome student?

- If an auditor called in to handle a receivership you'll heighten anxiety and find people unco-operative.

- Selling life insurance . . . projecting security in purple is difficult.

- At your first luncheon as an executive wife if you want to 'fit in' not 'stick out'.

- When you are depressed, it will make you feel more depressed.

COLOUR VITAMIN | GREY

Includes: Mid-tone shades to charcoal plus pewter, pearl and taupe (grey/beige).

Psychological Power of Grey
Positive Attributes: Respectable, neutral, balanced.
Negative Attributes: Non-commital, deceptive, uncertain, safe.

Wearing Grey for Emotional and Physical Impact
- In business, greys are the safest options for suits. Less authoritarian than navy or black, greys present a smart, professional look while being the least memorable.

- Team-up with a strong accent, such as a red, violet or salmon blouse, to project innovation and creativity while still being professional.

- For a job interview, but only with your seasonal white, if you need to play it really safe.

- Acting as arbitrator in any sort of dispute – major or minor.

- When wishing to project a balanced, unbiased attitude.

When to Avoid Wearing Grey
- On any occasion when you wish to be noticed, in grey you will fade into the woodwork.

- On dates which you hope will lead to a marriage proposal. If you wear grey too often he'll be scared you'll turn him down!

- In the creative sectors, except for meetings with traditional clients; even then, use one of your bright colours for a blouse or scarf.

- If working with children – they need to know where you stand at all times and grey will make them anxious. (Children respond best to primary colours.)

- When you need to be a catalyst, to make things happen; grey will hold you back.

COLOUR VITAMIN **| BLACK**

Black is the absence of colour due to the total absorption of light.

Psychological Power of Black
Positive Attributes: Formal, sophisticated, mysterious, strong.
Negative Attributes: Mournful, aloof, negative, lifeless.

Wearing Black for Emotional and Physical Impact
- As a sign of respect particularly in bereavement but also in cultures with different social and moral attitudes towards women (for example, in Muslim countries).

- For bold impact and contrast with one other colour, as when wearing a black skirt and red jacket.

- To keep people at a distance; we don't readily approach someone dressed in black.

- In the evening, for dinner parties or formal occasions, if your objective is to play safe and not stand out. The little black dress may be the easiest option but it doesn't enhance your chances of being noticed unless it's in your seasonal palette.

- If it's in your season, for lingerie in the finest fabric you can afford and the most alluring design to compliment your body.

When to Avoid Wearing Black
- If you enjoy people and like them to open-up to you; especially true if dealing with the elderly or children.

- At a wedding, black is sombre, stately not joyous.

- Near your face unless you have the strength of natural colouring to handle it

(OK for Deep Autumns, Winters, Clear Springs). Otherwise plan to spend at least an hour making-up to look alive.

- On television, it's an instant decapitator and appears heavy. Viewers' eyes are drawn down from your face to what you are wearing.

- If you haven't much time for personal grooming; black shows every speck of dust, cat hair and piece of fluff.

COLOUR VITAMIN ▌ WHITE

Colour produced by the reflection of visible rays of sunlight.

Includes: Pure, soft white and ivory shades.

Psychological Power of White
Positive Attributes: Pure, clean, fresh, futuristic.
Negative Attributes: Clinical, 'colourless', cold, neutral.

Wearing White for Emotional and Physical Impact
- There is a strong association of white with traditional medicine. So, if the objective is to project impeccable standards of care and hygiene white will do it (provided it is always clean).

- To create strong contrast against dark shades, such as navy, charcoal or black, which projects authority (the pseudo-policewoman effect).

- As a first-time bride.

- All over for an attention-grabbing, progressive image.

When to Avoid Wearing White

- If you have minimal time for personal grooming, as it shows every mark.

- As a complete outfit in the evening, unless you're near the equator and want to look and feel cool.

- In grubby urban areas where anything white requires daily laundering.

CHOOSING VITAMINS FOR THE DAY AHEAD

Every morning you should open the wardrobe and let your senses guide you instinctively. How do you feel? Are you full of life and optimism? If so be careful about wearing your brightest colours as you may overwhelm people all day long. When tired and listless at the start of the day, or when you're feeling 'blue', the last thing you need to wear is navy. Opt instead for some spicy shades or yellow or green to boost your confidence.

After considering your mood there are other factors to consider before you select your colour vitamins.

- **Will you be in the spotlight?** Or can you fade into the woodwork? If attending an important meeting, presenting or attempting to command an audience's attention you need the strongest, brightest colours in your palette.

- **Practical considerations** Darker colours are always more serviceable than light ones, but medium to light tones can be very effective provided you aren't a natural attractor of dirt.

- **Individuality** Some colours express great individuality and personality. You can use your wardrobe to be unique or to conform. We all have days when we need to do one or the other.

- **Symbolic messages** Do socialists and conservatives always want to show the flag by wearing red or blue respectively? Do you want to express your concern for the environment by wearing your greens?

Maybe there are colours you never wear. Red often is cited by many women as something they steer clear of, and some people consider green to be bad luck. An aversion to brown or grey may be due to bad associations with grim school days and a hated uniform.

If you've never worn one of these colours but you are now going to give it a try, begin to do so in moderation. The professional woman who has an important presentation pending may decide a dose of red is required. But if you've never worn red before, you'd be best advised to try some red in a blouse or as a pocket handkerchief rather than a whole red suit. Otherwise your adrenalin will run rampant and you'll forget what you're talking about. As you become more familiar with colours and how to use them you can dare to use your colours as vitamins in larger doses: the bold yellow jacket, the white suit, orange jumpsuit or purple evening gown. The decision will be to balance what makes you *look* as well as *feel* your best.

Improving your assets

COLOUR is only part of the challenge in selecting clothes that will make you look your best and help you project a successful personal style. You also need to understand what cuts, fabrics, patterns, textures, and proportions compliment you.

Think about your favourite skirt. Why does it always look good and feel comfortable? Why does a certain dress always bring you compliments? One thing is for sure, your best styles aren't necessarily the most expensive hanging in your wardrobe; they might even have been bargains that were chosen by chance but have become trusted friends that you turn to again and again.

If you analyse the design, fabric and details of these favourite clothes you'll start to get an idea of what styles suit you. Similarly, if you have clothes that never look or feel right, so that even if you try them on again after weeks of neglect, you hurriedly remove them – ask yourself, why? Is it the colour, the cut, the cloth or all three?

Interpreting Fashion for Yourself

Even when it's clear why your favourite things are winners, you won't want to be limited just to wearing those fabrics and shapes, and you need not be. With a good basic understanding of what shapes, proportions, length, fabrics and details suit you, you will be able to interpret any new fashion idea. Women of any age, whether 16 or 60 plus, can enjoy fashion and look up-to-date.

Looking current does not mean having to spend a lot of money on new clothes every season. No, if you have an understanding of what looks good on you, all you do each season is to add one or two new pieces to update your favourites in keeping with your lifestyle and budget. It's easy, the CMB way.

Essential Details

To understand what styles suit you, we need to analyse your:

● **Body shape**: How angular or how curvy are you, and what should be emphasised?

- **Proportions**: How balanced is your body; where are you long or short?
- **Height and Bone Structure**: Are you petite, average or grand in scale?

This information will help you to understand why certain skirts, trousers, jackets, and so on really suit you, and guide you when trying new styles to add more variety to your look. Once you learn how to identify and how to compliment your own personal body shape, proportions, height, bone structure and face shape, you'll be able to interpret new fashion ideas with confidence.

Forget the Scales

Weight is not a major issue in assessing your body shape. Extra pounds won't change the fact that you are, for example, either Angular or Curvy. But if you are an Angular body shape you will 'soften' as you gain weight and will need some easing of your basically crisp designs.

Think of Elizabeth Taylor. In recent years she's fluctuated from a size 6 to a size 16. But even when she is very slim, she is still curvy, and if she puts on weight she still has an hour-glass figure – albeit more rounded and less defined. The point is that she can never be angular, and therefore is not suited to crisp, severe designs. Her build is essentially soft and curved.

Why was Princess Diana's wedding dress a disappointment and the Duchess of York's such a success? Diana was ill-advised to bury her elegant lines under layers of excessive flounce. She looked lost. Fergie, by contrast, has a more rounded figure, and looked terrific in the soft gathers and nipped-in waist.

Your body shape is determined by your bone structure and the distribution of muscle and fat around it. Your shape can be altered through exercise, hormone imbalance, age, and of course, pregnancy and cosmetic surgery. But most of us stay essentially the same basic shape from late teens onwards.

ILLUSION DRESSING

After years of advising women of every shape and size I can assure you that to look your best you don't necessarily need to lose weight. However, you *do* need to come to terms with who you are and accept yourself. Why try to become what the fashion industry projects as an ideal figure, when that is constantly changing anyway? Sometimes they would like us to believe that we should be pin-straight, almost boyish in figure, then the full-figured 'hourglass' is *de rigueur* once again. Life is too short to waste it on wishing we had longer legs, a fuller bust, narrower waist or whatever. The only reason your weight should be a concern is if it affects your health and your ability to enjoy life.

Instead of wishing you were different, concentrate on making the most of what you have and learn how to 'balance' your figure by implementing a few clever tricks that we image consultants use every day. We've learned to play up our assets, and to minimise our liabilities. Now it's your chance to learn how to do the same. Let me introduce CMB's guide to discovering your body shape along with advice on how to make the most of your natural assets.

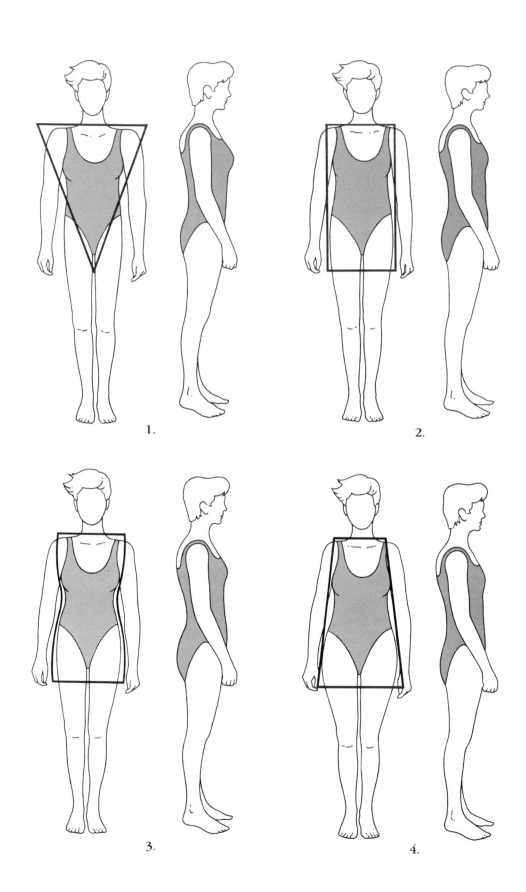

1.

2.

3.

4.

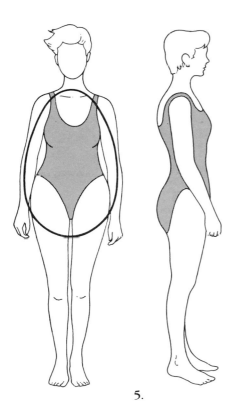

5.

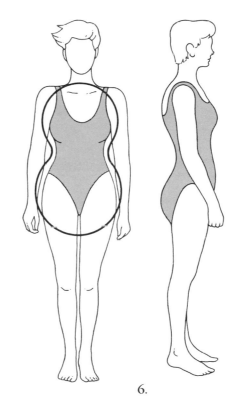

6.

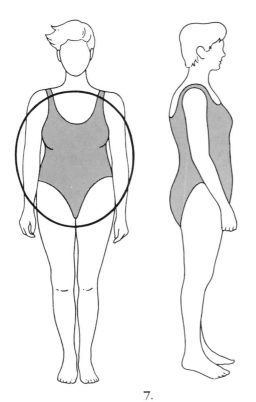

7.

Your Body Shape

Bodies seem to come in all shapes and sizes, but they can be identified within this range of basic body types, which extends from the very angular woman (with shoulders wider than her hips), through to the woman who is straight (with fairly even hip and shoulder measurements), to the 'pear' and 'hourglass' figures (who can be angular or curvy) and, finally, to the soft, rounded woman.

1. **Inverted Triangle**
2. **Straight**
3. **Softened Straight**
4. **Angular Pear**
5. **Curved Pear**
6. **Hourglass**
7. **Round**

What shape are you?

How do you determine which of the seven body shapes shown on the previous pages is yours? First you need to assess your silhouette, the outline of your body, from a front as well as a side perspective. This is best done wearing minimal clothing (a swimsuit or leotard is fine) and looking into a full-length mirror. First study your frontal reflection carefully. Where is the emphasis?

- How straight, rounded or sloping are your shoulders? Slightly sloping shoulders suggest a Curved Pear, while soft and rounded shoulders suggest a Round body shape.

- Are your shoulders narrower than your hips? If so, consider the Angular Pear or Curved Pear shape.

- Is your waist clearly defined or pretty much in line with your hips? Put your hands on your waist, at the sides, then move them down along the sides of your hips. Are your hands rounded as you move from your defined waist over rounded hips? Or is your waist in line with your hips?

- Are your hips flat or curvy? Curved hips suggest a Curved Pear, Hourglass or Round body shape.

Now turn sideways. Where's the emphasis? All women have defined bust lines and bottoms but how pronounced are yours?

- If your bust is larger than your hips, consider the Inverted Triangle shape.

- If your bust is smaller than your hips, the Pear is more you.

How curved and pronounced is your bottom?

- Flat bottoms indicate a straight/angular frame.

- Curved bottoms suggest a Pear, Hourglass, Softened Straight or Round shape.

Let's look at each shape in detail to help you decide which basic figure type is nearest to yours. For each type I have suggested a well-known personality who shares the same characteristics. Some of these may surprise you! That's because these women are usually practised in the gentle art of illusion dressing and appear to onlookers to have no figure faults. You too can achieve this effect. All you need to know are the best clothing styles for your figure shape.

The Inverted Triangle Shape

The Inverted Triangle comes in two variations. First, there are very angular women with boyish or athletic figures whose shoulders are broader than their hips. Many of these women have 'created' this look through exercise; Princess Stephanie of Monaco and Grace Jones are two examples.

The other version is the broad-shouldered 'top heavy' woman, whose bust is larger than her hips, and her hips and bottom are flat, not curvy. Victoria Principal is a good example.

The Inverted Triangle looks best in sharp, crisp styles. Since your shoulders already create a dramatic impression don't accentuate them any further with shoulder pads or epaulettes. If your bust is full, keep details in that area to a minimum.

Your broad, straight shoulders need balancing with your narrower bottom half. To do this, keep the texture in your fabrics tightly woven and crisp for blouses, tops and jackets. Looser weaves will tend to make you look broader.

The Inverted Triangle will want to compliment her figure with simple designs and use colour rather than pattern for effect. Fussy prints take away from your dramatic lines, as do gathers at the waist, which make you look heavy. You look striking in a simple jacket with a straight skirt or leggings.

Because the Inverted Triangular shape is often an athletic build, these women can show off their legs in short lengths or with interesting details in their hems, such as kick pleats, gored skirts or contrasting trim. Since her top half dominates her figure, a low heel or flat shoe compliments this woman best.

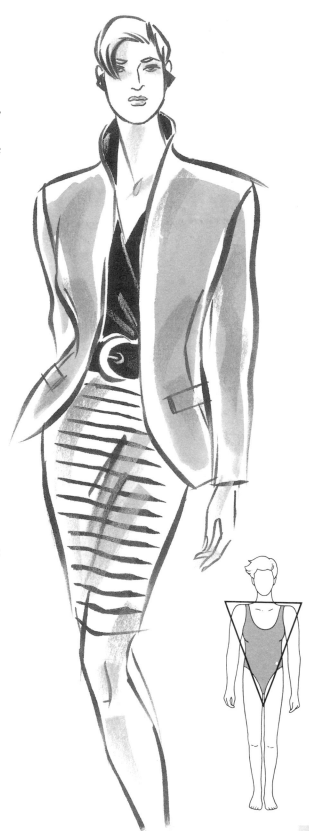

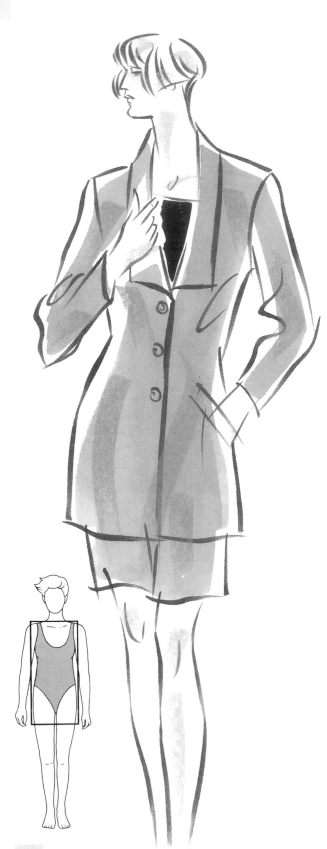

Straight Body Shape

From the front profile, this body shape has shoulders and hips pretty much in line. The waist is not more than 6 inches (15 cm) or so less than her hip measurement. If you think you belong to this type, place your hands on your hips and slide them down. They will feel flat, that is, your hands won't curve from your waist over your hips.

Straight Body shapes come in slim and ample models. Princess Diana is Straight Body type, and so, too, is the comedienne, Victoria Wood.

Look at your side profile. If your bottom is flat you are probably a Straight Body type. If your back curves and your bottom is rounded you will be in the Softened Straight category.

The Straight Body type looks good in tightly woven fabrics, like wool gaberdine, linen and Thai silk, and in sharply-structured as well as unstructured designs. The trick is not to make too much of the waist area. Jackets or dresses that contour in at the waist, but not exaggeratedly so, will be fine.

Your flat hips and bottom mean you will be best suited by waistlines (on skirts and trousers) that have minimal, if any, gathers. Opt for straight darts instead. Pressed down pleats are also good.

If you are exceptionally underweight and have a straight body type, follow the above advice but add layers to create bulk and give you a healthy as well as an interesting look. Skimpy, tight, straight designs on a very slim body are unsuccessful.

Sleeves are best kept straight, tapered and crisp. The set-in sleeve will feel most comfortable and create a straight shoulder line that compliments your build.

The Softened Straight Shape

This is a modified version of the Straight Body type, having the same straight shoulder line but a more defined waist. Princess Caroline of Monaco has square shoulders but her small waist means she looks most exciting when she wears softer skirts. Madonna is a Softened Straight Body type too.

While the Softened Straight shape follows much of the advice on fabric and cut given for the Straight Body type, she can make more of her defined waist. Belts are her key accessory. The greater difference between her waist and hips – 7 inches (18 cm) or more – means she will need a little more easing in her waistlines for skirts and trousers, with inverted pleats and soft gathers used in moderation (at the sides of the tummy) for best results. The sarong style is great on her.

Unlike her curved counterpart she will keep fabrics, designs and cuts more defined. Tight to moderately woven weaves are better than very loose ones which won't make the most of her essentially straight lines. Double-knits in simple neat designs are great on the softened Straight shape, as is wool crêpe for suits or dresses. Jersey fabrics in simple cuts without too much volume are also flattering as they allow both definition (at the waist where you want it) and movement – important for all women where they are curvy.

For jackets, fitted cuts make the most of a Softened Straight Body but if you like more relaxed designs, the simple, unstructured jacket nipped in with a belt or left open to show off your waist is a good option.

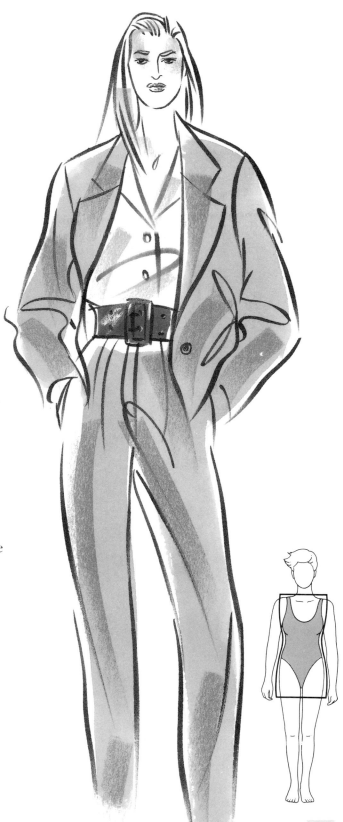

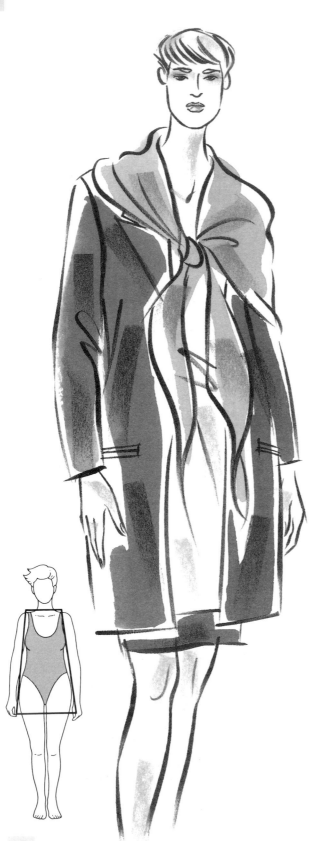

The Angular Pear Shape

Narrow at the shoulders and broad on the hips describes the traditional Pear shape, but there are both Angular and Curved variations.

The Angular Pear shape has narrow shoulders but they will still be straight, not sloping. From the side profile her tummy and bottom are flat. Her hips, running down to the thighs, are also straight and flat. Penelope Keith and Nancy Reagan are good examples of this traditional pear, who look better in simple designs than in excessive flounces and gathers.

The key accessories for any pear shape are shoulder pads, to balance shoulders with hips.

The Angular Pear will use straight shoulder pads not curved ones and to be current they won't be exaggerated. Other tricks for extending the shoulder line include wearing puffed or pleated sleeves, epaulettes, or shawls and scarves over the shoulders. Peaked or pointed lapels on jackets also create a widening effect.

Follow advice on fabric and details given for the Softened Straight Body Type but you will need even more easing at the waist. You've probably already learned to put up with the fact that all your skirts and trousers will be loose on the waist in order to fit over your more ample hips. Never opt for the reverse – a neater fit at the waist at the price of great strain over the hips. Be prepared rather to spend a bit of time or money on having the excess at the waist tapered for a proper fit.

To help create a balanced shape, select jackets the same size as your bottom (provided they don't hang off your shoulders too much). Also layering works to create more volume on top where you require it.

The Curved Pear Shape

Like your angular counterpart you, too, are smaller on the top and broader on the hips. The key differences is that your silhouette from front and side is more curved. The Duchess of York and Meryl Streep are good examples of this shape.

From the front, if your shoulders are curved or sloping, and if when running your hands from your waist over your hips you feel more rounded than flat, then you are the Curved Pear shape.

You, too, need to balance your figure with shoulder pads but choose curved designs, not very square ones.

From looking at your profile you'll notice that your bottom is rounded. This will need easing at the waistline with soft pleats or gathers. Beware not to choose styles with gathers running completely around the waist as this would make you look bigger than you are.

Boat necklines create a widening illusion at the shoulders. Draping crossover necklines, when generous in cut, give you some softness to compliment and balance your figure. Avoid slim-fitting tops which accentuate the difference between your upper and bottom half.

Your best fabrics are softer, more loosely woven than the previous Straight Body Types. For example, wool crêpe, jersey and challis give you welcome ease. Anything too crisp will make you look heavier than you actually are.

As a more curved body type, your patterns should be soft; for example, florals, curved abstracts, paisleys, etc.

The advice for the following two Curved Body Types will also be relevant.

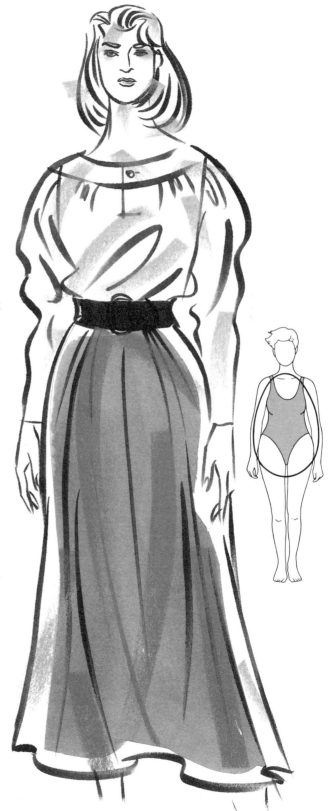

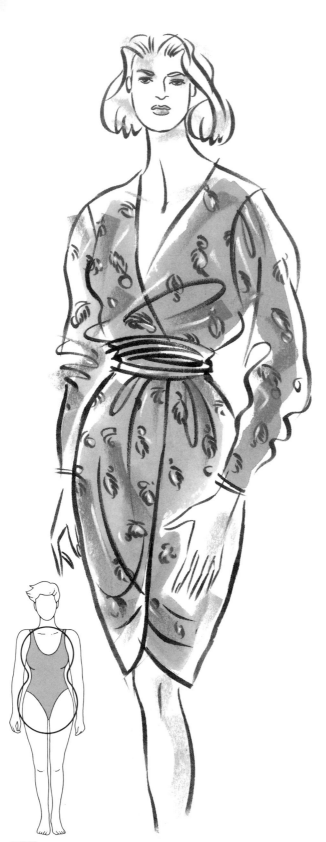

The Hourglass Shape

Here we have men's ultimate fantasy figure and the one that's envied by many women. But the Hourglass shape also has its challenges, as those who have it well know. For example, it is very difficult to find professional looking suits or dresses for this body shape.

From the front and side profiles you see curves. The shoulder line is soft, the waist defined, the hips rounded, the bottom and bust pronounced (not necessarily large) and curved. Both Paula Yates and Dolly Parton have Hourglass shapes.

The Hourglass must be careful with both design and fabric. The cut of her clothes needs to be soft, gathered and eased. She should avoid set-in sleeves (unless in a soft fabric) and opt instead for gathered, raglan or eased shapes. The lapels of jackets should not be sharp but rounded, such as a shawl collar. Her necklines are draped, round, crossover, or ruffled. Her pleats are soft, not crisp.

She must accentuate the waist – which is at least 10 inches (25 cm) smaller than the hips. If she doesn't, she will look larger than she is. Her waistlines will always be eased, as her hips are curved. Straight darts or restricted waistlines will make her look fat.

The full-busted Hourglass should beware of loose, baggy tops which can make her look frumpy and larger than she really is.

Like her Curved Pear and Rounded counterparts, the Hourglass selects soft designs such as florals, polka dots, paisleys and soft abstracts. These are far more flattering over her curves than stripes or plaids.

Round Body Shape

The Round Body shape is probably an overweight Curved Hourglass. When Elizabeth Taylor gained all her weight in the early 1980s she moved from an Hourglass to a Round Shape. The Round Body Shape needs to keep her look loose and unstructured, never tight and defined. She should always make sure she buys clothes in a size large enough to get the proper fit. Roseanne Barr is another example of this shape.

If this is your shape, like the Straight Body type you will want to avoid attention at the waistline. Longer jackets and drop waistlines are the most attractive. Happily rounded comedienne Dawn French shows how terrific the overscale longer jumper, teamed with leggings, can look on this body shape. Emphasise your shoulderline which should be the focus from which all your styles lead. Tops, jackets and dresses should drop in a simple unstructured straight line from the shoulder. Beware of too much draping, texture, fabric and pattern as they will make you look heavier than you are.

Shoulder pads can be a big help to balance your top half with your lower half. Easing at the waist is essential, with soft gathers or pleats giving you the movement you need. Long over-blouses, sweaters and jackets are slimming when teamed with skirts.

The Rounded Body shape is often short-waisted, but this usually means there is extra leg area to play up. Skirts cut on the bias or softer culottes with longer jackets take the eye away from your broadest point – the middle.

Emphasising your neckline with soft collars, attractive necklaces and scarves will also help to divert the attention from your middle and direct it to where you want it – on your face.

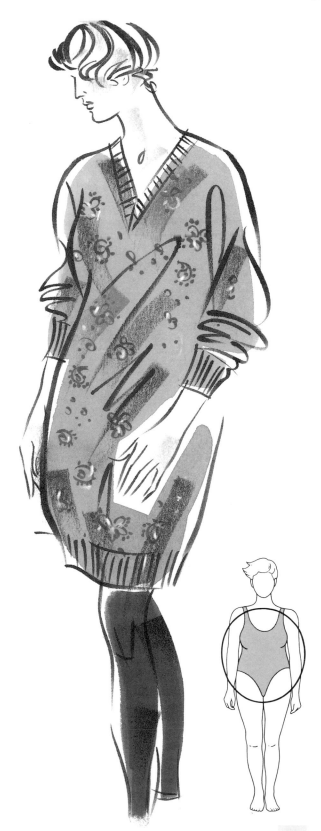

THE BALANCED BODY

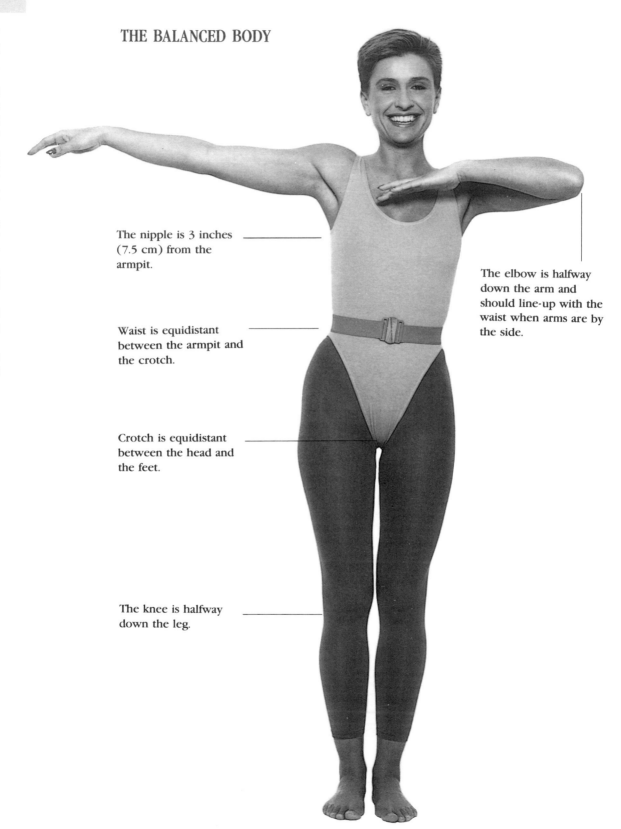

The nipple is 3 inches (7.5 cm) from the armpit.

The elbow is halfway down the arm and should line-up with the waist when arms are by the side.

Waist is equidistant between the armpit and the crotch.

Crotch is equidistant between the head and the feet.

The knee is halfway down the leg.

PROPORTIONS

Have you ever wondered why some styles make you look thicker in the waist than others, and why some jackets are fine and others make you look like a squashed mushroom? Or do you get frustrated when shopping with a friend, who wears the same size as you but looks terrific in long skirts while you look dreadful in them?

The answer is your 'proportions'; that is, the distribution of space from head to toe. Some of us have long torsos, others rather short ones. Some have short legs, while others have legs that seem to go on and on.

Unlike your weight or muscle tone, you can do nothing to physically alter the proportions you were born with. The challenge is to learn how to deal with your particular proportions and to learn what styles, lengths and cuts are most flattering for you. Once you learn the following easy but effective tricks you will be able to adapt current fashions so that they work for you – whatever your proportions.

How evenly proportioned are you?

A good way to discover your proportions is to stand in front of a full length mirror, barefoot and in your undies, then mark your height, and the positions of shoulder, armpit, waist and crotch on the mirror with an old lipstick. If you find this awkward to do yourself, ask a friend to mark the key points.

The Waist/Torso

If your upper half and bottom half are evenly balanced, your crotch will be half way up your height (that is, equidistant between the top of your head and the floor). Similarly, a balanced waist should fall halfway between your armpit and your crotch. If your waist is above half-way, you are short-waisted; if it is below the half-way mark, you're long-waisted.

The Legs

If your legs are evenly proportioned, your knees should measure half way between the floor and the 'break of the leg' (bend your leg and you will see the point, below the hip, where the leg 'breaks'). If they are long above the knee you will have more choice in skirt lengths.

If you have been 'short-changed' somewhere in your proportions you will be 'compensated' somewhere else. For example, if you are short in the waist, you will be proportionately longer in the legs. If given a nice long waist area, alas, you will have been short-shrifted in the length of your legs.

The good news is that any unevenness in proportions can be balanced and even turned into an asset, once you know how to complement your proportions with the styles you wear.

Long Legs/Short Torso

Let's focus first on the plus part of your proportions; that is, on your long legs. You are the one for whom those beautiful long skirts are made: where you have the length you want to create the interest. Skirts cut on the bias, gored, with kick pleats, knife pleats, long sarongs or culottes are all designed just for you, as are skirts with detailed hemlines. If you are short-waisted, mid-calf lengths can succeed only when you balance them with short cropped jackets, so giving the illusion of longer legs.

If you like short skirts, however, there's no reason why you should not wear them. Just remember that you already have a lot of leg on show so don't go too far above the knee; mid-thigh styles on you can look very daring.

Avoid wearing high heeled shoes as these would make your legs look out of balance with the rest of your body. Choose low heels or flat shoes instead.

Create interest by your choice of hosiery. Toned-in with your hemline is most elegant, but you can also consider patterned designs to make the most of your long limbs. Your goal is to draw the attention to your lower half – and to your face, of course – and away from your shorter mid-section.

A shorter torso needs only a few tricks to create the illusion of more length. First avoid deep belts or any kind of fuss at the waistline. Longer jackets 'lengthen' the torso area and can make you look thinner at the same time. Soft, unstructured jackets ending mid-thigh (provided your hips are not too broad) or going down to the knee, are great.

Dropwaisted dresses, overblouses, large blouson sweaters (especially worn with leggings) and low-slung hip belts all help to lengthen the waist area and visually balance your proportions.

Short Legs/Long Torso

You want all the action in your upper half, in your torso, where you have more length, so create the attention at or above the waist. Belts are your most important accessory; be as bold as you want – depending upon how trim your waist is.

Change boring buttons on your jackets, substituting more interesting ones to attract attention and visually 'break-up' your long torso. Short jackets, of bolero to hip length are best.

To lengthen your short legs, just remember that shorter skirts are best – from just above the knee to the mini, depending on muscle tone, age and whether they are appropriate wear. If you prefer longer skirts, be sure still to show plenty of leg. Even when the fashion might be ankle length skirts, you will need to keep your skirts above mid-calf to look well-proportioned.

Choose your hosiery to tone with your skirt and shoes; avoid light or patterned hose which draws too much attention to your short legs. Always aim to create a lengthening illusion.

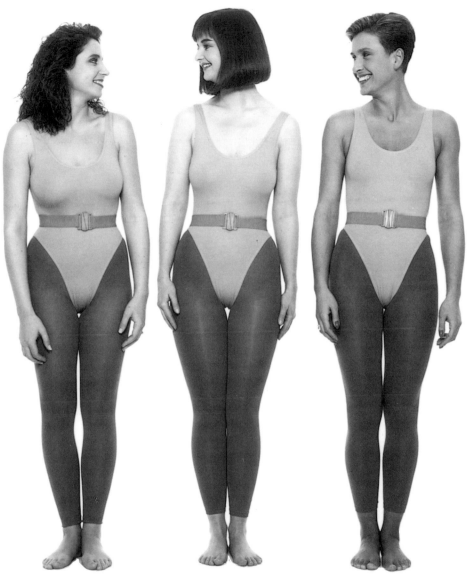

Short-waisted figure

If you are like Lisa, above, your waist will be short but you are wonderfully long-legged. You need to draw attention away from your waist to those lovely legs. See page 84 for how Lisa achieved this.

Long-waisted figure

If you are like Sarah, above, there will be lots of room for belts and features at the waist – your best asset. However you are short in the legs. Turn to page 85 to see one of Sarah's best looks.

Balanced figure

This figure has the widest options when selecting flattering styles to wear. See page 80 to find out whether you, like Joanna, have a balanced figure.

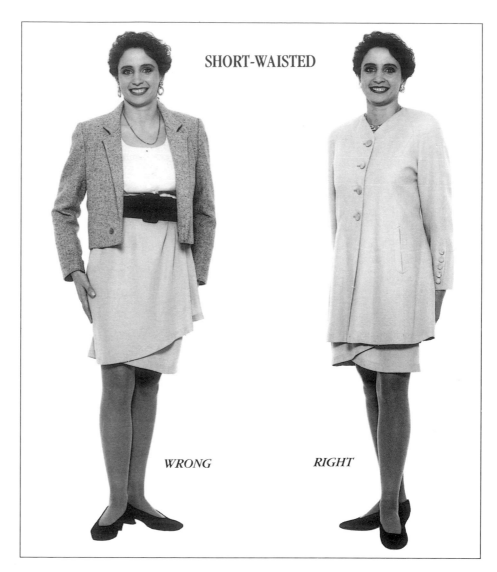

SHORT-WAISTED

WRONG   *RIGHT*

Wrong

Lisa has a short waist and should avoid short, cropped bolero-style jackets like this one, in preference for longer styles. Wide or contrasting belts create clutter in the waist area where there isn't a lot of space. So if you have a short waist, select belts that are modest in width and tone them in with the colour you are wearing.

Short skirts are terrific on any woman with legs as nice as Lisa's. But beware if you have long legs and show much more than this, as you can look scandalous. Long skirts are terrific on you.

Right

Lisa is wearing the same skirt but a different jacket. Notice how slimming the effect becomes when Lisa lengthens the line. Removing the clutter from her waist makes her appearance more balanced.

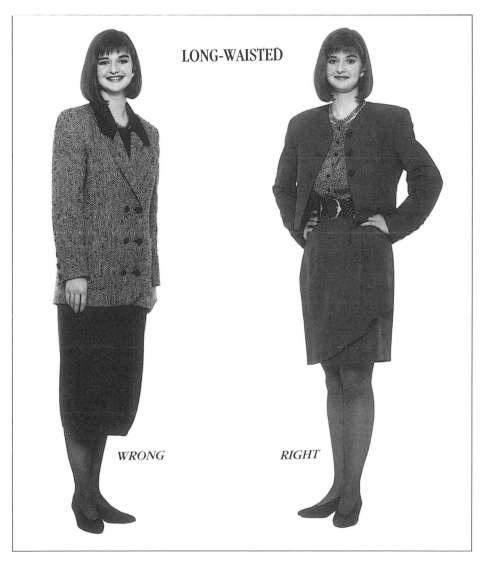

LONG-WAISTED

WRONG   *RIGHT*

Wrong

Sarah is a striking 5 foot 8 inches (1.7 m) with a long waist; however her legs and arms are short for her stature. The length of the skirt, i.e. mid-calf, when teamed with this jacket, does nothing for Sarah. Her best bet will always be shorter skirts.

Right

Short jackets bring the attention to the waist area where there is room for wide belts. Choose them in contrasting colours, or to match the bottom half which gives a lengthening illusion. Loose, boxy styles are terrific on the long waisted, but also consider fitted waists with belts or gathers. If you like long jackets, choose seven eighths or nine tenths proportions and wear with a short skirt just peeking out from the bottom. A long jacket with a long skirt will make you look shorter.

HEIGHT/BONE STRUCTURE

Along with getting the proportions right, you need to understand the significance of height and bone structure in developing style. Think for a minute about your sweaters. You might own both finely woven tight knits and loosely woven, nubby designs. Which type feels more comfortable? Do the neat knits make you look bigger? Do those large, loosely woven styles look and feel more comfortable? Or, when you wear that overscaled, fuzzy sweater do you feel dwarfed, whereas the finer knits make you feel better?

The right amount of texture and the types of weave we look best in depend on our bone structure and height, as well as our body shape. Some of us have big bones, others are very fine or small boned; some are just average. Measure your wrist to find out the scale of your bones; do this over your wristbone. You will probably find it easier to let someone else do it for you.

Fine Bones	5½ inches (14 cm) or less
Medium Bones	5½–6½ inches (14–16 cm)
Grand Bones	6½ inches plus (16 cm plus)

Next let's look at your height to see if you are small, medium or grand scale.

Petite	Under 5 feet 3 inches (1.6 m)	Small scale
Average	5 feet 3 inches–5 feet 6 inches (1.6 m–1.65 m)	Medium scale
Tall	Over 5 feet 6 inches (1.65 m)	Grand scale

Putting it Together

If you measured Grand Bones and Scale, you can wear more texture and larger prints than smaller women. But we've worked with many tall women who had average or even fine bones. They have to be careful not to go over the top with the large prints and very bold accessories which many tall women wear so beautifully. The answer is to find the right balance. If these tall, fine-boned women wear small-scale designs (such as a tiny floral print) these will only make them look taller. You can see this effect on our tall model, Anna, on page 88.

Conversely, petite women with Fine Bones know that it's easy to look overwhelmed by wearing prints that are too bulky or heavy for their small frame. The large print dress worn by our petite model, Teoh, on page 89, completely overwhelms her.

Everything from fabrics to accessories – your earrings, belts, handbags, and shoes – should be in proportion to your Small Scale.

However, if you are a petite woman and have Medium to Grand Bones you need to add a little more texture, so choose slightly stronger prints and wear chunkier accessories to look balanced.

Opposite: Teoh and Anna back to back.

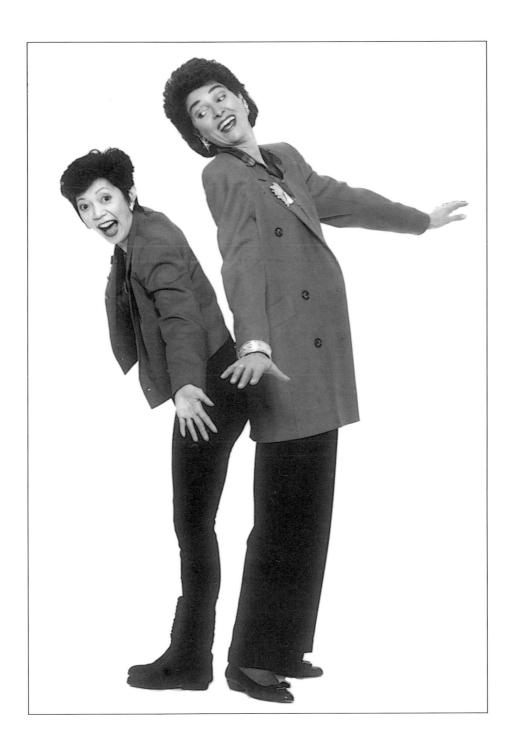

Test Your Scale

Now that you know whether your scale is Small, Medium or Grand, spend some time in a department store just trying on new possibilities. Compare different size earrings, belts, handbags, shawls, and try some of them with your outfit. You'll find the difference they make to your overall look very apparent.

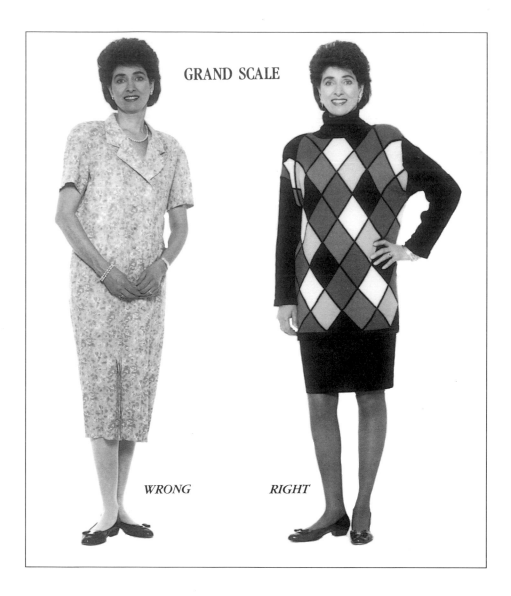

GRAND SCALE

WRONG   *RIGHT*

ANNA

Wrong

Tall women, like Anna, make themselves look larger than life when they dress in small prints and use accessories that are too insignificant for their dramatic scale.

Right

Go for it! Anna's striking stature demands larger, bolder designs. Only Grand Scale women can wear these with success.

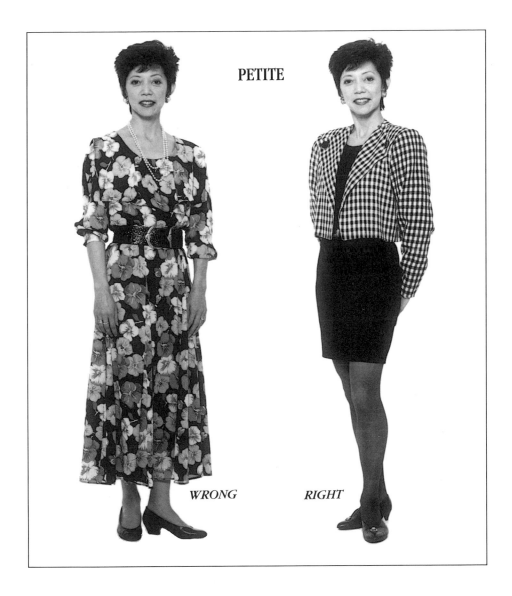

PETITE

WRONG *RIGHT*

TEOH

Wrong

Petite women need to take care in choosing prints. Medium to large scale designs can look overwhelming, the result unsuccessful. This dress fits Teoh but the pattern swamps her. She looks like a little lady in a big dress.

Right

It's better to use prints in moderation when you are petite, for example in a jacket on its own or a scarf over a plain top. You draw attention to your face when you use prints creatively on the top half.

COLOUR TRICKS

You can use colour, too, to draw attention to certain areas and features and to distract from others. Certain colours recede and are slow to catch attention, whilst others jump out and catch the eye.

The first place you want to draw attention to is your face, the centre of communication with others, the mirror of your personality. Accepting that you will be wearing make-up that enhances your natural colouring, I want you to concentrate on the colours you wear on your upper half (above the waist). The colours of your blouses, sweaters, scarves and jackets reflect most immediately and directly on to your face. Choose favourite shades from your seasonal palette when making your first investments to team up with more indifferent colours you might already own for skirts or trousers (the bottom half).

Light colours such as pastels and white 'advance'. If you wear these on your lower half, you can appear larger than you are. Darker shades have the opposite effect, they 'recede' and can give the illusion that you are smaller. But beware of the ill-founded adage that black makes you look slimmer. If you wear black all-over for this reason and it's not in your seasonal palette you will look pale and tired, and focus will be drawn down to your body, to the colour which is overpowering you – exactly where you *don't* want attention.

A bright contrasting belt draws attention to your waist, so if yours is trim and a real asset, belts are definitely for you. Bold coloured hosiery will also attract attention, so be sure your legs merit it before you buy bright shades.

Colour can enhance or exacerbate your scale. If you are petite and wear separate blocks of colour in a jacket, blouse, skirt and hosiery, you 'break' yourself up into smaller bits which can make you look much shorter than if you wear tones of one colour all over. Try the one-colour dress or toning blouse and skirt with a different jacket for good effect. If petite, always tone your hosiery with the colour of your skirt and shoes to 'lengthen' your legs.

Tall women have a longer length to work with so they can be more adventurous in using several different blocks of colour. If you are tall, the contrasting blouse and skirt with a complementary jacket will help to condense the impact of your height. If, however, you want to emphasise your powerful stature, all-over tones of one colour will make you appear even taller than you are. Perhaps the easiest way to create interest and break-up your length is to use a smart, contrasting belt and/or hosiery (lighter than your hemline).

BALANCING ACTS

As you have seen, most figure challenges can be overcome with a few, simple balancing strategies. It you are short in an area, e.g. the waist, you keep it uncluttered so it appears longer, more balanced. For areas you can't balance, you can camouflage. Shoulder pads may not be in fashion, but they can transform women with sloping shoulders into looking taller and slimmer.

Now, here is CMB's quick reference guide to help you maximise your assets and minimise your liabilities.

CHALLENGE	WHAT TO AVOID	WHAT TO LOOK FOR
Long necks	Open, plunging or bare necklines. Long chains exacerbate the effect as do short-cropped hairstyles.	High, stand-up collars. If worn open, fill with a choker or scarf. Hairstyles that are long and full are best.
Short necks	High collars, e.g. polo, mandarin, cowl or excessive clutter with scarves or necklaces. Long hairstyles tend to emphasise the problem.	Open necks: V, boat or jewel necklines if face is angular; draped, scooped or crossover if face is soft. Shorter hairstyles angled at the back give on illusion of length.
Thick necks	Rounded necklines and short necklaces. Scarves create unnecessary clutter.	Revers or open collars worn up; narrow V-necks.
Broad shoulders	Shoulder pads; unnecessary details, such as epaulettes; boat or strapless necklines.	Raglan or dolman sleeves; V-necks; long necklaces to break horizontal line of shoulders.
Sloping or too narrow shoulders	Dolman or raglan sleeves; strapless, deep or narrow V-necklines	Shoulder pads, epaulettes, puffed sleeves. Boat-shaped or slashed necklines.
Long Arms	$3/4$ length sleeves or ones just above the wrist. Anything too tightly fitted.	Short, capped sleeves, wide cuffs. Pile on the bracelets, if appropriate.
Short Arms	Sleeves longer than wrist bone; capped or short. Excessive cuffs, particularly in contrasting colour. Baggy sleeves or unnecessary bracelets.	Sleeves $3/4$ length, pushed or rolled up. No longer than wrist bone.

CHALLENGE	WHAT TO AVOID	WHAT TO LOOK FOR
Small Bust	Open or deep necklines. Clingy or tight tops.	Extra details like pockets, lapels; interesting patterns; horizontal designs. Layers and a loose fit create the illusion of more generous curves.
Big Bust	High neckline and collars, excessive details and trim such as pockets; short sleeves; cropped jackets; highwaisted skirts; tightly cinched waists, contrasting belts.	Open and V-necklines; shoulder pads or broad shoulder designs. Generous draping on the top. Drop waistline in dresses. Over-blouses. Moderate size belts same colour as the top.
Long-Waisted	Long jackets, e.g. $^3/_4$ length, drop waists, belts in the same colour as top.	Cropped, bolero jackets or $^7/_8$ or $^9/_{10}$ lengths that just skim the skirt. Wide belts if waist allows, same colour as the bottom. Empire/high waistlines look terrific.
Short-Waisted	Cropped, bolero, short jackets; high-waisted trousers and skirts, wide belts.	Longer jackets (ending below hip line); drop-waisted dresses; over-blouses; narrow belts same colour as top.
Wide Hips	Gathered, full pleated waistlines; stiff tight fabric; details in pattern or design on hips, such as pockets.	Either longer line jackets or short styles avoiding the hip area depending on your proportions. Soft easing at the waist to the side of tummy but not gathers over hip area. Centre seam skirts help narrow the illusion.

CHALLENGE	WHAT TO AVOID	WHAT TO LOOK FOR
Broad Bottom	Shorts, trousers, straight tight skirts; short, fitted jackets.	Skirts with ease at the waist and loose (not full) over the bottom. Longer jackets that end below the bottom; blouson or unstructured best. Bring attention to your upper half through use of colour.
Heavy Thighs	Tight or short skirts, leggings, or shorts.	Softly gathered waistlines for skirts and trousers. Culottes can be both comfortable and flattering.
Heavy Legs	Short skirts, contrasting, coloured, light or textured hosiery. Flat shoes.	Longer skirts that end at the natural indentation below the knee or tea length (i.e. just above the ankle) – depending upon height. Tone hosiery to match shoes, and best if medium to dark (but not opaque). Simple shoes with a slight heel.
Skinny Legs	Short skirts, contrasting or coloured hosiery. Stiletto heels.	Longer skirts or culottes. Lighter tone hosiery will make legs look fuller but should tone with hemline or shoe. Low or flat heels best.
Short Legs	Long or full skirts, wide trousers, palazzo pants, turn-ups. Flat shoes or stiletto heels. Long jackets.	Monochromatic, blends of colour or one overall colour. Tone hosiery with hemline and shoes. Low to medium heels best. Shorter skirts (depending on your legs), shorts, cropped trousers, short jackets.

chapter six . . . .

The finishing touches

THERE is little point in spending time, effort and money on building a terrific wardrobe of flattering, co-ordinating clothes if you are going to neglect the finishing touches. Attention to make-up, hair and personal grooming is vital.

MAKE-UP POLISH

When relaxing at home, at weekends or on holiday, it's great to give the skin and yourself a break from wearing make-up. But otherwise, all women look and feel better with a little colour, 'their' colours, to enhance their skintone, eyes and hair.

If you hate the idea of wearing foundation, or feel 'too obvious' in any make-up at all, you're probably using the wrong products as well as the wrong shades. Cosmetics today are light and easy to apply, with good quality products to be found in every price range. And they are much more natural looking than they used to be.

In corporate image seminars I show women how to achieve an effective, natural, professional make-up in just 10 minutes each day. If you follow the seven steps given below, you'll only need to touch up your powder and lipstick to look fresh for eight hours or more!

Need I add that you should always start with a scrupulously clean face – and a light moisturiser if you have dry skin. Seat yourself in front of a well-lit mirror–daylight is better than artificial light.

Step 1: Concealer

Many of us have shadows on our faces which make us look tired and drawn, even if we've had a good night's sleep. Shading comes with age (starting in the late twenties) and can appear around the eyes because of vitamin deficiencies, general neglect or a stressful lifestyle. In some cases it can be hereditary.

Take a look at where there are dark patches, areas or lines on your face. We'll begin by lightening these to blend in with the rest of your skintone.

- To use as a concealer, choose a foundation lighter than your skintone, and dot on lightly in those shaded areas. Allow the foundation to 'settle' for a minute, then begin blending it in – gently – using your ring finger (this is the finger that has the most delicate touch).

- For darker circles and shadows use a thicker foundation or concealer in an even lighter shade, and cover the area completely. Apply with a soft, natural bristle brush, a foam applicator or your ring finger.

Step 2: Foundation

Don't be tempted to skip foundation; without this base the rest of your make-up won't last more than one hour. Also, foundation helps to even the tone and texture of your skin. Just as an artist prepares her canvas before painting, using a neutral 'wash' for a base on which to be creative with colour, so must you provide a smooth, receptive base for your make-up.

- Choose a colour by testing shades along the jawline. You want one that blends in, rather than being distinctive.

- The best way to apply foundation is with a foam sponge. Put a small amount on the back of your hand, take up a little of this at a time on to the sponge and apply evenly, in downward strokes, all over your face and lips but not your eyelids. Take particular care to blend in well along the jawline as you do not want an obvious line, but do not take the foundation down and over your neck.

Step 3: Powder

A complete dusting of translucent powder (avoid the eyes) is now necessary to 'set' the foundation so that it will last all day. Never apply powder blusher directly on to a cream foundation because it will not blend in softly; your skin will 'grab' it and look blotchy and harsh.

- Choose a translucent powder that is 'colourless' or neutral in shade, so that it blends with your skintone.

- Apply powder all over the face with a large, fluffy brush, dusting across the forehead and down over the cheeks, nose and across the mouth, chin and jawline.

- Alternatively, press in using a powder puff to set the foundation completely. Oily and combination skins are advised to do this rather than use a brush which may not be as effective for your more moist skin.

Step 4: Blusher

Blusher enhances your bone structure and gives you a natural healthy glow; that is, if you choose the right shade (see your Seasonal Palette for ideas).

Powder blushers are longer lasting than cream. But if you find they 'disappear' on you, try using a cream blusher after foundation (before powder), then dust with a powder blusher to enhance the colour and your chances of it lasting longer.

Apply blusher along the base of your cheekbone, from mid-cheek up to your hairline, brushing it on with short, feather strokes and going right up to the hairline. Don't overload the brush and avoid going too high on the cheekbone or into the middle of your face.

Step 5: Eye Make-up

- Use a dab of eyebase cream to lightly cover your lids and orbital bone before applying any colour. This will help to keep your eye make-up fresh all day, without creasing or running. You also need to use less shadow when it is applied over a base.

- Dust all over the eyelid and orbital bone with a light neutral shade of eyeshadow, like peach, soft pink, lemon or champagne.

- Eyeliner helps define your eyes and make your lashes look thick and rich even if they are actually a bit sparse. Kohl pencils create a softer effect. They are best used only on the outer third of the upper and bottom lids, which helps to 'widen' the eyes. Choose a colour which compliments your eyes (consult your Seasonal Palette). Black is too harsh for most eyes and inappropriate in business.

- 'Set' the kohl liner by brushing lightly with a powder eyeshadow along the line. A short bristle brush is best to dab powder along the lines of the upper and lower lids. The colour doesn't have to be the same as the liner; you can create many different effects by experimenting with various colours of powder on top of different kohl pencil liners.

- On the upper lid, work from the eyeliner in upward strokes applying a smoky, rich neutral to the outer third of the lid. Sweep from the outside of the orbital bone inwards. Brown, grey, aubergine, navy or moss green are excellent for adding depth and look polished, not artificial. Avoid bright or pearlised shades for work. Save these for when you want your eyes to sparkle in the evening. Keep colours within your Seasonal Palette.

- Finish with mascara on the top lashes at least. Use netural browns, greys or dark navy. Bright coloured mascara is too distracting and takes attention away from your eyes.

Step 6: Eyebrows

Your eyebrows frame your eyes, the centre of our attention, so make sure they do your eyes justice. Consider the attention you would give to framing a special picture or painting. The same care is needed for your eyebrows.

If they are sparse, fill-in with soft, feathery strokes of a sharp pencil or dot in eyeshadow of a neutral brown or grey – just a shade lighter than your natural brows. Finish by brushing upwards with a clear mascara to give them even more life and texture.

Step 7: The Lips

The tricks for achieving long lasting lipstick are to:

- Apply lipstick over foundation and powder. Choose a colour recommended for your Season.

- Opt for matt lipsticks with strong pigments rather than glossy or very pastel lipsticks.

- Use a lip pencil in a natural shade to outline as well as fill in the lips. Then apply your lipstick over this. Because a pencil is more waxy it lasts longer than lipstick and gives you a colour-base to last all day.

- You can apply lipstick straight from the tube or use a lipbrush. Afterwards blot with a tissue, then reapply lightly.

GROOMING ESSENTIALS

Regardless of income, background or lifestyle, modern women have no excuse for being badly groomed. We can all transform our appearance simply by bothering to attend to details – and a little regular care and attention doesn't take as much time as you might think. Here are some guidelines.

Hair

Clean, conditioned and well-cut. Individual needs obviously vary but, at minimum, have your hair trimmed every 6–8 weeks.

Skin

Cleansed, moisturised and protected. Develop a basic skin care regime. There is no need for expensive facial treatments. Once a week expose your face to a bowl of steaming water to open pores and cleanse away built up grime. Add herbs to the steam for an added treat. Try lavender or camomile.

Eyebrows

Well-shaped and tidy. Pluck regularly as necessary.

Teeth

Brushed and flossed at least twice daily. Try to brush after lunch as well to ensure fresh breath. Have your teeth professionally checked and cleaned at least twice yearly.

Breath

Bad breath has something to do with how regularly you brush and floss your teeth but more often than not the problem connects with the level of acidity in your system due to eating and drinking patterns, and tooth or gum decay. If halitosis *is* a problem, try to cut out coffee and tea (except herbal varieties), alcohol and acidic foods. Each morning, drink a glass of water containing a pinch of bicarbonate of soda, to counteract an acidic system and keep your breath fresh. If you think or know that your gums are the problem, consult your dentist without delay. Modern dentistry is quick, efficient – and painless – so why put up with unnecessary social embarrassment and the risk of losing teeth?

Body Care

Skin care for the body is not an indulgence, it's a necessity to keep you looking toned, fresh and well-groomed. Just as the face needs regular deep cleansing and moisturising, so too does your body. Use a natural bristle brush, loofah, body scrub or body mitt made for rubbing vigorously over the body to remove dead skin. Do this when the skin is dry. Moisturise your body with virgin olive oil weekly, rubbed into your damp skin after a warm shower (use about a dessertspoon of oil on a moistened flannel).

Body Odour

Body odour can be caused by the foods you eat (curry, Mexican food, cheese) or by wearing stale clothes. Aside from the obvious safeguard of bathing regularly (that is, daily), appreciate that odour often comes from new sweat mixing with old sweat on clothes. Be sure that your clothes are dry cleaned or laundered and aired regularly to prevent any unpleasant odour. Also use a deodorant if your system is acidic and omits an unpleasant odour. Most natural sweat, off a fresh clean body, is quite pleasant.

For women who perspire heavily a deodorant won't prevent wet underarms and clothes; an anti-perspirant/deodorant is what's required. However, women who don't have overactive sweat glands should stick to using a simple deodorant as natural sweating helps to flush out toxins from your system.

Facial Hair

I know, life isn't fair. Some of us are darker and fuzzier in places we wish we

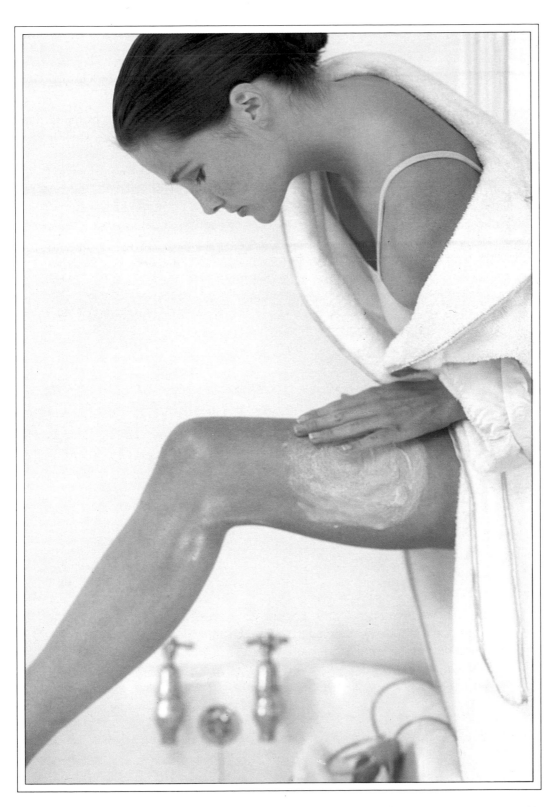

A couple of times a week use a body scrub, bristle brush, loofah or body mitt to polish up your skin

weren't, and during our period a female 'moustache' can become darker and more noticeable.

If you have noticeable hairs on your face you have three options:

- Bleaching them monthly. This is fine if the hairs aren't coarse or too long. Apply a special facial hair bleach to lighten the hair. Follow the manufacturer's instructions. Always test a patch of hair on your arm first. Some women's hair turns red, which can be worse than the natural shade.

- Using a depilatory, a chemical that dissolves unwanted hair. These are available as creams, gels and sprays. Make sure you use one formulated especially for the face. Try a patch test initially to be sure you won't react to the chemical.

- Having electrolysis, which is the only method that permanently removes hair. It can be a slow, time-consuming and expensive process but it's the best long term solution to an embarrassing problem. Only qualified professionals can perform electrolysis; they insert into the hair follicle a fine needle through which an electric current is charged to kill the hair root. Fine hairs need only one session; stronger coarser hairs may need several treatments before they disappear permanently.

Legs

Most people agree that leg hair that is dark, long or stubbly is not attractive and needs regular treatment. There are three viable options:

- Shaving

- Using a depilatory

- Waxing.

Any one of these three options are fine provided you do it regularly. Electrolysis is a huge undertaking which proves far too expensive and time-consuming for most busy women.

Bare legs have their place on holiday or at home or on relaxed social occasions, but for working women, the change to a warmer season is no excuse for abandoning tights. To avoid discomfort on really hot days wear stockings to help with ventilation, and avoid those using Lycra (which allows little, if any, 'breathing'). Another option for working women is to travel to and from the office bare-legged, but wear tights or stockings whilst working.

Hands and Nails

You use your hands all day long to express yourself. Think of how aware you are of other people's hands and ask yourself what impression yours give. You can't do anything about the shape of your fingers or the size of your hands but you can enhance them tremendously through regular and simple grooming, including the maintenance of nails and cuticles and by using hand cream or lotion to keep the skin soft and smooth.

Keep hand cream or lotion at every sink where you wash your hands and carry a cuticle cream and emery board in your handbag for regular touch-ups.

To have beautiful hands and nails a weekly manicure is a must. But don't panic, it is very easy to do this yourself. Consult an assistant on a department store beauty counter or treat yourself to a professional manicure and watch how it's done. I find doing it at a set time each week is the best way to ensure it gets done.

HAIR, YOUR CROWNING GLORY

Hair is something women universally complain about. 'If only it were a different colour/had curls/was straight/thicker/or shiny.' We have all had the experience of the disaster cut, the one that made you look like you were wearing somebody else's hair. You wondered how you could possible live with it. That whimsical 'new look' takes months to grow back into something more recognisable, more comforting, more you.

Choosing a good hairstyle requires two things. First you need to know what will suit you: your face, your lifestyle, and, most importantly, the type of hair you have. Secondly, you need the help of a talented yet sympathetic stylist.

Face Shape

If yours is a simple oval shape there'll be lots of possibilities within the limits of the texture of your hair. For women with other shaped faces – square, oblong, round, etc – you are advised not to repeat the shape of your face but to create complementary width, softness or length where you need it.

For example, oblong faces will be emphasised and appear even longer with straight styles that end at the shoulder or below. It's better to 'break-up' the extra length of these faces with angular or soft styles that create width at the sides and back.

Square faces, by contrast, have more width and less length than oblong faces. So opt for the minimum on the sides with layers on top to create height, and some length showing at the back to create length.

In selecting a style to complement your face, you will achieve a more balanced and interesting look. A lovely round face that has a full, round hairstyle just looks fat, not interesting. You make the most of your face by choosing a hairstyle that shows off its own uniqueness.

Lifestyle

If you are unlikely to spend a half hour every day working with your hair it's fruitless to choose styles that require a lot of care and crimping. Longer styles can be time-consuming if left free, but if attractively plaited, pulled-back or up can be as easy to care for as some of the shorter styles. Before choosing any new look be sure to discuss with your hairdresser how much time you want to spend daily in caring for your hairstyle.

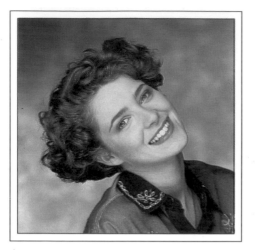

1. ●

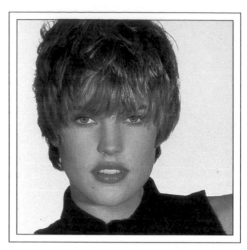

2. ●

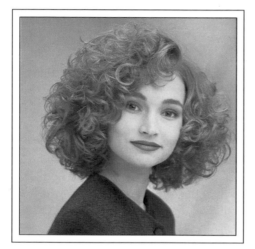

3. ●

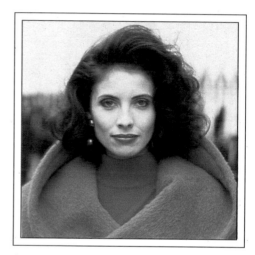

4. ●●

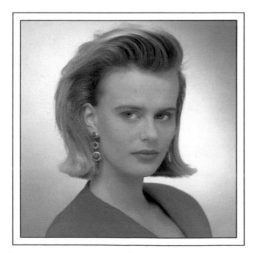

5. ●●

1. For naturally curly or permed hair. Great for all face shapes except those with a wide forehead.

2. A terrific cut for hair of all textures except very thick. Can be worn smooth, parted, scrunched or allowed to fall naturally into a striking fringe.

3. For naturally curly or permed hair. Fills out oblong faces and those with a wide forehead. Best avoided if you have a square or round face.

4. Hair of average thickness required for this style, as well as with some body. If hair is fine consider a body perm or jetting to achieve fullness. Great on most face shapes except square.

5. For fine to medium thick hair. Good for oval and round faces.

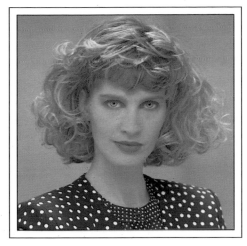

6. ●●

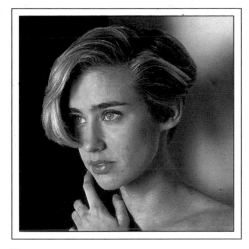

7. ●●

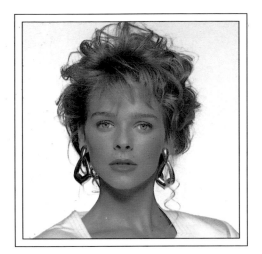

8. ●●

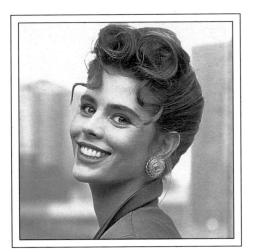

9. ●●●

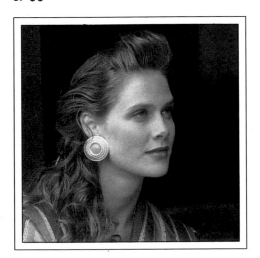

10. ●●●

6. Volume like this on medium length hair requires a lot of mousse after drying hair with head bent forward. For natural, body-waved or permed hair.

7. A modern cut for busy women. Avoid only if you have a long neck.

8. Medium length hair loosely pinned packed in a clip. A great way to transform your look for the evening.

9. Average to long length hair with medium to thick texture. A stunning style for most face shapes except the oblong.

10. Long full hair for the woman with lots of time. Avoid if you are petite or average height – best on tall women.

(For key to symbols see page 104)

Texture

How thick or thin your hair is and how much body it has (on its own without mousses or gels) will affect your choice of styles. While you might hanker after the luscious locks of particular magazine models or your best friend, they may have a different *type* of hair to yours, and you'd be smarter to learn more about making the most of your own hair, and how to look *your* best.

On pages 102–103 are some styles for you to consider. Each is captioned with its suitability for different face shapes and hair texture, and is coded for effort (● wash and wear; ●● blow-dry necessary; ●●● time required for tonging, rollers or other fiddling).

Choosing Your Stylist

Look for a stylist who falls somewhere between the bland, uninspired yes-person who will do whatever you tell him/her to do without offering constructive advice, and the dictatorial hairdresser who insists on creating whatever he/she wants with little if any involvement from you. The best hairdressers are sympathetic as well as creative. They need to listen to what you envisage before telling you what's possible.

Many hairdressers will debunk the photo you have torn from a glossy magazine that shows the look you want. But a good stylist should take a look at it to get a sense of your desired image. They should then advise you whether or not such a look will be possible with your hair, and if so whether it will suit you. Remember that what we see in the magazines is often the result of hours of work using all sorts of gels, mousses, rollers, pins, even hair pieces, to create the effect. So use pictures in magazines as a guide for a new length, colour, or image rather than trying to copy a look exactly.

Here are some useful tips to help you succeed with hairdressers:

- **Dress the part**   You appearance dictates how the stylist interprets your image. So don't pop in, unplanned, in your jogging suit, unmade-up (unless that's your daily look) and then expect them to give you anything chic.

- **Demand discussion**   Don't settle for the cursory 30 second size-up. Take whatever time is required before your hair is washed to discuss your ideas, and get all your questions answered about the possibilities.

- **Ask lots of questions, observe**   If seeing a new stylist or getting a new look, be sure you know what will be involved with creating the look yourself. If mousse or gel is required, when do you apply it – before or after blow-drying, or both? What's the best method of blow-drying – with your fingers or using a hairbrush? What sort of hairbrush? If you wanted to create something else with your style, what are the possibilities? Don't expect your hairdresser to actually create all the other looks, but you do deserve the time to be talked through ideas for using combs or bands, pulling back, making fuller with hot rollers or tongs, etc.

- **Never make an appointment for a Saturday** Your hairdresser has probably been out on the town on Friday night and so won't be up to par. Also, Saturday hairdressing is an assembly-line operation. Stylists have little time to devote to discussion and are probably fully-booked and always running over time. A stressed and hurried hairdresser can be lethal.

- **Change your hairdresser every once in a while** Your favourite stylist gets used to seeing you in a certain way and might not be the best one to advise you on a new look. Once you've tried something new you can return to your former stylist and explain you had it done when away on holiday or business. If you like it tell him/her so and why. They'll get the message that the new you is happy and wants to maintain the current look and not return to the former one.

- **Choosing by referral** If looking for a new hairdresser ask women (whose hair you admire) who does it for them. All women love to receive a compliment and should be delighted to share the person behind their mane. Shop assistants in fashion stores or behind the beauty counter will happily proffer their hairdresser. These women are in the beauty business and are used to sharing tips with other women.

TIPS FOR COLOURING YOUR HAIR

Today women have a multitude of choices for treatments to enhance their own natural hair colour. And why not? In Britain, where regular sunshine is in short supply, many natural blondes can look rather muddy and lifeless unless they highlight their hair. But any CMB seasonal type can colour her hair provided she follows guidelines that will ensure best results. Should you go too far with a new hair colour you can weaken the effect of your Seasonal Palette. I'm not saying don't ever try something different, just beware that you may need to adjust your seasonal colours if you do so.

Let's consider the available techniques, before looking at some guidelines for each Season. The various options come down to a choice between temporary and permanent colour. If you haven't coloured your hair before, it's better to try out a new shade with a semi-permanent or shampoo rinse to see if you like it. A permanent tint or bleached highlighting is a serious commitment that will take months to grow out.

Temporary Colour
You can begin to test various shades with coloured mousses or shampoo rinses. These only coat the surface of the hair and wash out with your next shampoo. Women with dark hair will find it difficult to judge the results as these treatments don't show up as effectively as on light-haired women.

Semi-permanent Colour
You can experiment by selecting a colour off the shelf, but I would advise you to seek the help of a colourist in a good salon. Don't expect every hairdresser to advise you accurately on colour. A specialist is required to tell you what's

possible with your hair, that is, how porous it is and how it is likely to take colour. A specialist will also be able to tell you which colours will complement your skintone.

Semi-permanent colours are shampooed into your hair and left for about 20 minutes before rinsing out. For best results, shampoo your hair twice before applying, as the cleanest hair is the most porous.

Semi-permanent colour is only advised for red, auburn, brown or dark hair as it really isn't effective as a lightening treatment. Try a semi-permanent colour if you are just starting to go grey as the natural fading won't be as obvious as with an all-over permanent tint.

Semi-permanent colour lasts up to six weeks, fading gradually back to your own natural shade with no obvious difference between the tint and your own hair colour.

Permanent Colour Tints

Here's the heavy-duty treatment of dyes mixed with hydrogen peroxide to permanently change the colour of your hair. You'll begin to notice re-growth in four to six weeks and will then need the roots to be dyed to blend in.

This is your best solution should you wish to change the colour of your hair significantly or to cover grey completely. Always go to a specialist for this treatment (see Semi-permanent Colour above).

Bleaching is the permanent colouring treatment if you want to go blonde. The time required depends on your hair type but results are certain.

Any permanent colouring affects the natural texture of your hair, making it both more porous and dry and susceptible to splitting. Be sure to treat your hair to a weekly waxing and use conditioner especially for colour treated hair.

Highlights and Low-lights

The half-way alternative to an all-over change of hair colour is to add 'lights'. Highlights are best for blondes and can be done ad hoc in different areas to create the effect of a few weeks in the sunshine. Dark and mid-tone brown hair is effectively treated with low-lights which streak in a shade richer than your natural colour to create interest and a sense of movement.

The benefits of professionally applied lights are that the results are very natural and the re-growth hardly discernible. Re-touching is required about every four months.

GUIDELINES ON HAIR COLOUR BY SEASON

Spring

Clear Springs: Choose chestnut or rich brown rinses, tints or low-lights. If greying nicely then leave, otherwise tint a colour slightly lighter than your natural colour.

Warm Springs: Red, strawberry or golden blonde lights work best. Add warm or golden highlights to grey hair.

Light Springs: If highlighting blonde use golden, not ash blonde highlights. Allow to grey naturally.

Summer

Light Summers: If blonde, select ash with some warmth. More neutral ash highlights are best if you also have grey. Beware of bleaching too platinum as it can be very ageing on the thirty-plus age group.

Cool Summers: You grey beautifully, so let nature run its course. But if you highlight your hair blonde, you'll need to switch palette to Light Summer.

Soft Summers: You will benefit from some highlights if your hair is a 'mousy' colour. Beware of going too golden. Medium ash highlights are most effective or low-lights in shades slightly lighter than your natural hair colour. Most Soft Summers grey attractively but will need to adjust their Palette to the Cool Summer colours when they do.

Autumn

Soft Autumns: Many Soft Autumns come to life with some extra colour from either high or low-lights. Opt for warmer, more golden highlights, not red or strawberry or you'll become a Warm Autumn. The effect of very warm colours on your skin is not successful so highlight carefully. Consider rinsing over the grey when it begins to appear (it will probably be an unflattering dishwater shade), or maintain your highlights.

Warm Autumns: Try strawberry or golden highlights. A semi-permanent henna tint is also very effective for Warm Autumns. When the grey appears you will have to decide whether to cover it. Alas it's not always flattering, so I recommend that you rinse it regularly with a shade softer than normal. If you don't cover the grey, adjust your colours to the Soft Autumn Palette.

Deep Autumns: Chestnut or auburn rinses or tints are best. If you use low-lights, you will soften your look and need to adjust your seasonal colour palette to a Soft Autumn. If you think you might be close to a Soft Autumn (eyes and skin wise) you can consider the switch. But if you are darker in skintone with a very strong eye, then don't lose your drama by going lighter. In most cases Deep Autumns don't grey attractively so rinse when the grey becomes abundant.

Winter

Deep Winters: Chestnut or auburn rinses or tints are best. Highlights will ruin the effect of your Seasonal Palette. Most Deep Winters grey beautifully.

Cool Winters: If hair is grey, I bet it's beautiful. Should you wish to colour it back closer to your natural hair colour you'll become a Deep Winter. But only do so if you are really keen. Your grey hair is a terrific asset.

Clear Winters: Keep deep and strong and close to your natural hair colour. Many Clear Winters grey beautifully. If you like it, go with it. Just remember that you'll need to soften your colours – when the grey becomes predominant – with the Cool Winter Palette.

GLASSES: THE EYES HAVE IT

If you wear glasses I hope you realise that they are your most important accessory. The same goes for sunglasses. Choose the wrong frames and you can look ineffective, unattractive and even sinister, but the right glasses focus all our attention on you and your eyes. Some women like to have several pairs so they can achieve different looks and there are some ideas for casual, business and evening looks on page 111. Other women find that one well-chosen pair is sufficient.

Selecting glasses can be a little daunting. Ophthalmologists are not trained in style and consequently aren't always particularly helpful when it comes to suggesting frame styles, colour or treatments that can enhance your face. Fortunately, you can easily learn the basics about selecting glasses as an accessory that enhances not detracts.

Colour Tips for Choosing Eyeglasses

Fashions come and go, so if you are opting for one pair of eyeglasses choose a good neutral colour that will compliment you and the type of clothes you wear.

For guidance look to your Seasonal Colour Palette (Chapter 3). Mid-tone neutrals, such as smokey grey, tortoiseshell, medium navy and olive (depending on which appear in your Palette) are best for workaday eyeframes. If your budget runs to a second pair, choose something more fun for weekends, that expresses both your seasonal colours and your Style Personality. A touch of diamanté will create 'after-six sparkle' for evening wear.

Complementing your Face Shape

In selecting glasses, choose frames that complement or contrast with the shape of your face – but don't repeat it. For example, round glasses on a round face would be uninteresting. Square glasses on a square, full face would be even worse, making the face appear wider and the jawline severe.

Here are some tips to help you when selecting frames:

Size
Select frames that are in proportion with your face. If petite you need more delicate styles; if you choose large frames you'll look dwarfed. The large faced woman needs more substantial frames; delicate ones would look too light-weight. Balance is the key.

Frames should be:

- no wider than the face
- in line with the eyebrows at the top
- no lower than the highest point of the nostril contour.

Narrow Faces   Rectangular or round frames are best; the aviator style is also good.

Square or Rectangular Faces   Choose frames with softened edges not angular ones. Square faces should avoid large frames – they look best if no lower than the top of the cheek.

Round Faces   Square or rectangular styles give definition.

Wide-set Eyes   Choose darker, stronger bridges which have the effect of bringing the eyes together.

Close-set Eyes   Select clear or narrow bridges which lighten the area and won't make the eyes seem even closer together.

Long Noses   Choose a low or dark bridge to shorten the nose.

Short Noses   A high or clear bridge make the most of a small nose.

Eye Make-up Tips for Spectacle Wearers

If you have poor vision this need not prevent you wearing eye make-up. Today there are glasses and aids to help you to do it with ease. Special, flip-down frames can enable you to see what you're doing one eye at a time. But magnifying mirrors are widely available to help any woman, no matter what the degree of myopia (near-sightedness) or hypermetropia (far-sightedness).

Far-sighted
The women who is far-sighted will have lenses that magnify the eyes. Hence, she needs to take particular care in applying eye make-up so that it doesn't look too exaggerated:

- Use neutral, natural tones. Bright, colourful shades will look brash and detract from the colour of your eyes.

- Use minimal eyeliner; on the outer third of the top and lower lid only. Avoid black altogether.

- Apply two thin coats of mascara rather than one thick one which could look clumpy.

- Keep any stray hairs under eyebrows trimmed, otherwise they will make your eyes look 'dirty'.

Short-sighted

Short-sighted women often have to wear lenses that make their eyes appear smaller. If this is your problem, you can minimise the effect in the following ways:

- Avoid very pale or pearlised eyeshadows. Use deep, natural shades to enhance the intensity of the eyes.

- Use a kohl pencil to line the eyes, to create definition and depth. Do not line the eyes completely as it makes them appear smaller, exacerbating your problem. Line only the outer half of the upper lids, and the outer third of the lower lid, to widen and deepen the eyes.

- Strengthen the definition of your eyebrows. If they are very light, brush in with a soft neutral shadow – similar to your own brow colour. Finish by brushing brows upwards with a clear mascara.

Colour Contacts

Contact lens wearers have a wide range of exciting choices with lenses that can enhance as well as transform their natural eye colour. The effects of coloured lenses can be subtle or striking but sometimes can look very bizarre and artificial.

Your eye colour is a key component of your seasonal colour analysis. If you change your natural brown eyes to blue you transform your whole look and the effects of your clothes and make-up. Should you plan a complete switch and expect to wear the new colour most of the time you'll need to adjust or even change your Season.

When you select tinted contact lenses to enhance your natural eye colour you create a brighter or deeper effect. The Soft Autumn's hazel eye, for example, when changed to emerald becomes more striking. Her Soft Autumn palette will now look bland and unexciting next to emerald. No doubt she'll need to become a Bright Spring in order to balance her look.

So consider coloured contacts lenses very carefully. I'd recommend tints to brighten or enhance the natural colour of your eyes rather than change their colour completely. But the choice is yours. Just remember you may be jeopardising your entire wardrobe for a whimsical challenge to Mother Nature.

Opposite: How to use different styles of frames

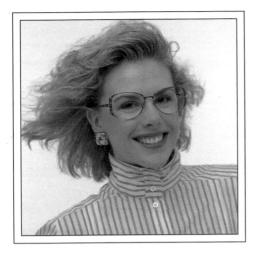

Casual

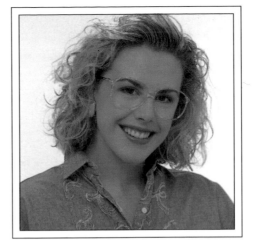

Casual

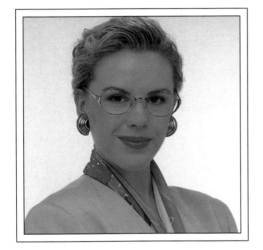

Business

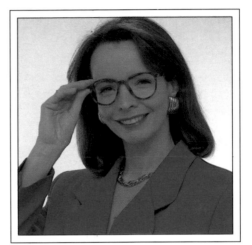

Business

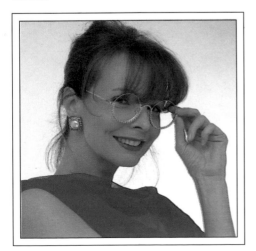

Evening

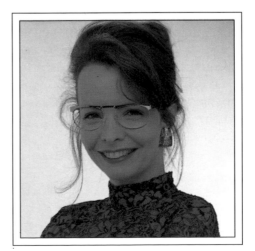

Evening

chapter seven

Style personality

NOW it's time for the inner you to come out and tell us how you want the world to view you. So far we've dealt with your physical characteristics – your natural colouring and your body shape – and you have learned a lot about what would suit you. But as you were discovering your colours you no doubt came across a few shades in your Palette to which you said 'Never in a million years.' As you read about your body shape, too, you might have gasped at a few style suggestions because you have either never tried them or just wouldn't be caught dead in them.

Your personality dictates your style, which is your own personal interpretation of fashion. If you ignore your personality and buy clothes influenced by glossy magazines or what looked terrific on a friend, you end up with a wardrobe that is a muddle of styles. This limits your flexibility in mixing and matching to create combination outfits, and means you are not getting the best value from your clothing investments.

I would not suggest for a minute that you should have a wardrobe of all the same fabrics, patterns and cuts. How boring that would be. But what I am advocating is that you analyse the fabrics, textures, prints, details and accessories you *like* the most, as well as which colours and styles suit you, and aim to build your wardrobe around these.

Your Many Moods, Your Various Occasions

Some days we feel carefree and want our look to reflect this. Other days we may be more reserved and perhaps even feel a bit beleaguered. On those occasions we don't want to wear either colours or styles that attract attention. Although we always want to look good.

Just as our moods vary, so do the social requirements of our lives. There are occasions, both special and routine, that call for different looks – days when we want or need to be dramatic, classic, natural, romantic, chic or creative.

Let's think about a sporty event, such as having a game of tennis with a friend.

Your partner might turn up in co-ordinated gear, with ruffles on her panties and socks, and – as she always does – wearing full make-up and perfectly coiffed hair. You could be wearing a comfortably over-sized T-shirt, outside your shorts for complete ease of movement, no make-up and with your hair functionally pulled back into a sensible pony tail. Or perhaps vice versa. Either way, two women will have brought two individual styles to the same occasion. 'Different strokes for different folks', and thank heavens for it; how tedious it would be if we all looked and dressed the same.

Think about how you dress for special dates with your favourite man. What did you wear on your most recent anniversary or the last time he wined and dined you? Was it a body hugging Lycra mini-dress or a lace blouse and long velvet skirt? Maybe your idea of dressing romantically is to don a jumpsuit not a dress. How we interpret our moods as well as different occasions is contingent upon our basic personalities.

When you dress in styles and accessories that reflect your personality we notice *you* first, then your clothes. You look and act yourself. When you feel at ease with your image you can be more relaxed, in any situation. In clothes that aren't 'us' we tend to feel contrived, 'dressed-up', self-conscious, or even silly. For any occasion, for any roles you perform, you can truly express your personality so that the focus of attention is *you*, not the designer's or your best friend's dress.

DISCOVER YOUR STYLE PERSONALITY

Take the personality test below. Tick the answer that most truly describes you; sometimes there may be two possibilities but choose the one you'd prefer. You might not know the famous women given as examples in Question 10. If this is the case, just leave that answer blank.

1. The type of clothes I prefer for work are:

A. Separates that mix and match, that are comfortable yet professional ☐
B. Classically-tailored suits ☐
C. Nothing too classic, preferably softer lines ☐
D. Fashionable, bold, powerful designs ☐
E. Appropriate but unexpected combinations ☐
F. Elegantly blended neutrals in the very best quality ☐

2. The type of clothes I prefer for weekends:

A. Sportswear or casual gear ☐
B. The timeless good-quality skirt and sweater ☐
C. Soft dresses, flowing skirts with pretty blouses ☐
D. Latest fashions, an overscaled jacket and striking accessories ☐

E. Ethnic, avant garde or unpredictable styles ☐

F. Simple but chic, like a designer tracksuit ☐

3. My favourite hairstyle is:

A. Casual, with a windblown, scrunched effect ☐

B. Controlled and neat but not severe ☐

C. Soft, full-layered curves, never short ☐

D. Sleek, asymmetrical ☐

E. Spiked, loose curls, or carefree ☐

F. Smooth styles that are both current and timeless ☐

4. My favourite fabrics are:

A. Viyella, denim, knits, texture ☐

B. Quality natural fabrics: 100% wool, cotton, silk ☐

C. Jersey, lace, silk ☐

D. Rich fabrics: velvet, brocade, suede ☐

E. Lycra, metallics, contrasting texture ☐

F. Best quality wool crêpe, cashmere, leather ☐

5. My favourite blouse or top is:

A. A wool or cotton polo ☐

B. Tailored silk or cotton ☐

C. A lace-collared blouse ☐

D. A bold overblouse ☐

E. A one-off design, very arty ☐

F. Jersey or stone-washed silk ☐

6. For accessories I choose:

A. Not much but preferably natural beads and stones ☐

B. Pearls or gold only ☐

C. Delicate pieces, preferably antique ☐

D. Bold, geometric shapes worn on their own – never jumbled ☐

E. Large drop earrings, ethnic pieces ☐

F. Gold ropes, Chanel-style earrings ☐

7. For evening, if I had my choice it would be:

A. Velvet trouser or jumpsuit ☐

B. Simple black dress ☐
C. A beautiful silk dress with fine details ☐
D. A colourful silk jacket with a black skirt ☐
E. Bicycle shorts and a sequinned top ☐
F. Smoking jacket, silk camisole and elegant trousers ☐

8. My favourite shoes are:

A. Trainers or ballet-style slippers ☐
B. Court shoes ☐
C. Higher heels, with open toes or sling-back ☐
D. Leather boots or striking 'statement' styles ☐
E. Short, suede 'shoe boots' ☐
F. Squared toe, wedged heel pump ☐

9. My favourite colours are:

A. Natural looking dyes, nothing neon ☐
B. Blended colours, never bold contrasts ☐
C. Pastels ☐
D. Rich bold colours against black ☐
E. From neon to ethnic ☐
F. Neutrals: charcoal, pewter, ivory or stone-washed shades ☐

10. I would like to develop a style personified by:

A. Anneka Rice, Jane Fonda ☐
B. Anna Ford, Princess Grace of Monaco ☐
C. Jane Seymour, Joan Collins ☐
D. Cher, Paloma Picasso ☐
E. Tina Turner, Madonna ☐
F. Selina Scott, Shakira Caine ☐

TOTALS: A's_____ B's_____ C's_____ D's_____ E's_____ F's_____

If you answered mainly: **A's** you are a Natural, **B's** a Classic, **C's** a Romantic, **D's** a Dramatic, **E's** a Creative, **F's** a EuroChic.

As with the previous chapters on colour and body shape, these Style Personality types are not absolute. You may be dominantly one type but have a strong second preference. Perhaps as a working woman you feel one way during the day but love to unleash a different you after work and at weekends.

To learn more about interpreting your Style Personality read the following sections describing your dominant type.

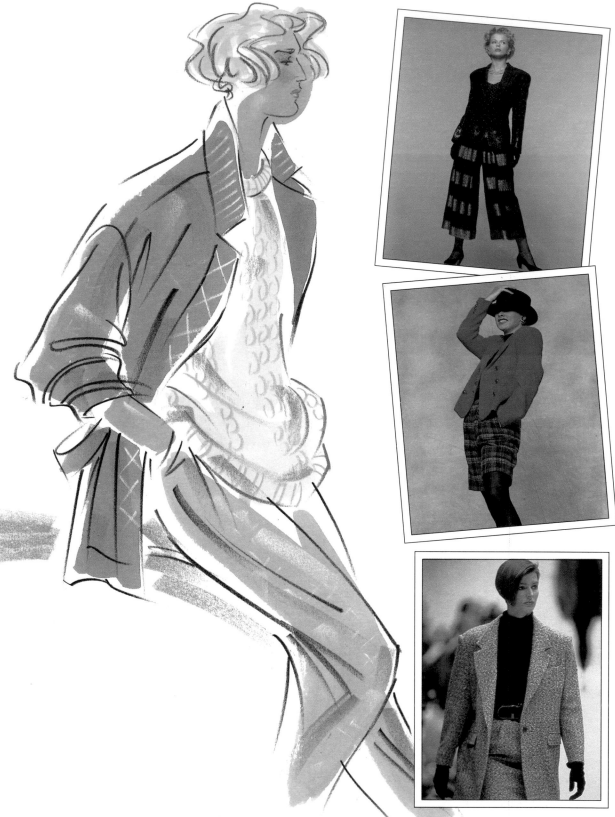

THE NATURAL TYPE

THE Natural Type has a relaxed style that begs ease of movement and fun. Out of the six types, you have the least interest in what might be fashionable. Your priorities are otherwise, but that's not to say you don't like looking good.

Your instinctive style draws you to nature, which inspires you most in your choice of colour. The Autumn Season has the most natural palette, but all CMB Seasonal Palettes have simple, uncontrived tones. Nothing neon for you: you are attracted more by vegetable dyes like sienna, ochre and indigo.

For prints, the Natural Type prefers paisleys, checks, plaids and stripes (provided they're not too bold). Anything too twee or too loud would make you fidget. You love texture and get away with the woolliest woollens and nubbiest fabrics. Your wardrobe mistakes will include frilly blouses, silk dresses and exaggerated designs.

Your styles require movement, so suits can't be too form-fitting and skirts must allow you a generous stride. Even though you might be slim you prefer eased waistlines. Inverted pleats or soft gathers give you the freedom you need.

Tips for Dressing Naturally

Colour   Nothing electric for a natural look; best are ecological tones: browns, russets, greens, yellow golds and hues from the sea – deep blues and sea-greens and sand. But all the Seasons can create a natural look. For best results, blend tones and add a flash of colour, perhaps in a scarf, collar or waistcoat.

Styles   Nothing too fitted, with enough room to layer. The Natural loves to pile on the layers, adding and subtracting as the weather dictates. Being an outdoor person, the Natural's clothes can't be too whimsical or unable to withstand the elements. Don't be lured by items you know you'll abuse, such as chiffon scarves or fine denier hosiery. Woollen shawls and opaque or ribbed tights are more your style.

Make-up   You like the bare minimum. But be honest, can you still afford to dash around in just a scrubbed face and a touch of lipstick? Try a tinted moisturiser (in your Season), neutral earth-tone eyeshadows, brown or black mascara and a natural lipstick or gloss.

Accessories   The natural style is best enhanced by accessories that are rich yet rustic. Handcrafted leathers and rough stone beads blend beautifully with suede, knits and corduroy. Your best investments would be a quality leather braided belt, bronze loop earrings and an antique-style stick pin for your lapel. For chains, choose nothing too shiny or delicate.

Hair   You don't want to devote too much time fussing with mousses, gels, hair-dryers or curlers in the morning. So choose a short style or a long one that looks wonderful when easily pulled up or back with a clip.

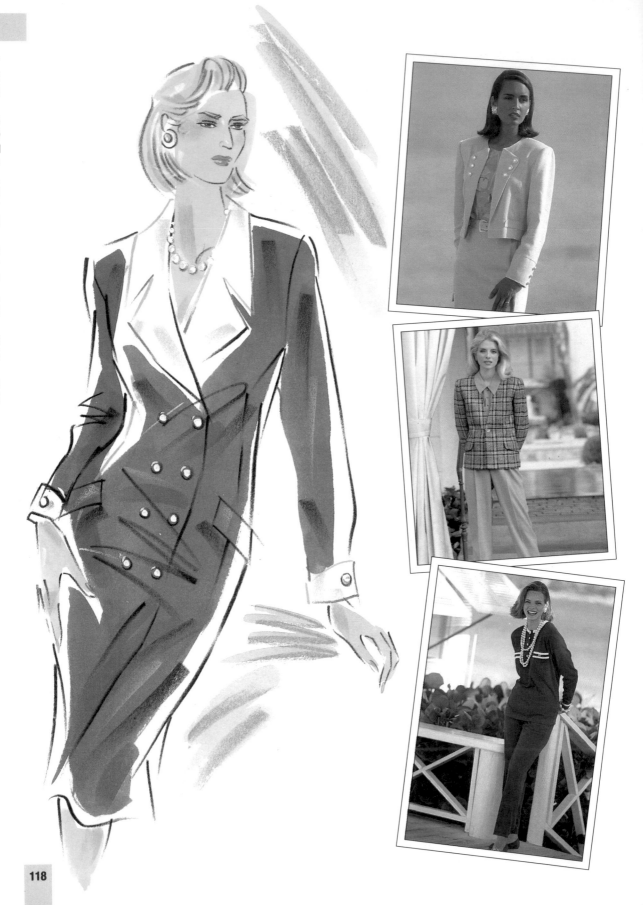

THE CLASSIC TYPE

THE timeless elegance of this style is best reflected by women who value quality more than quantity, style more than fashion.

You don't want your clothes to scream 'look at me'. Rather, they are understated. You like to blend your colours in a way that's never contrived.

Others who try wearing classic styles appear boring. As a real Classic Woman, you choose the most uncomplicated, simple designs and look superb. You can easily make a bargain dress look like a designer number simply by how you carry it – with that personal, graceful style of yours.

The fabrics you choose are never extreme; too much texture makes you feel uncomfortable. So rather than the large, overscale, bulky jumper preferred by the Natural Type, you always opt for the tightly woven, well-fitted sweater. Anything too fussy, frilly, silky or slippery is out; quality natural fibres are for you rather than the beaded, emboldened, trimmed or bedazzled anythings.

If you are a Classic Woman who sticks to her guns and remains unswayed by fashion trends or pressure, you can create a wardrobe that will take you anywhere. Your styles combine beautifully, so the business suit can easily and effectively be transformed for evening by a simple change of accessories.

Tips for Dressing Classically

Colour The mid-tones (blues, greens, purples) and the neutrals (cream, stone, mushroom, pewter and grey or brown) form the foundation of your wardrobe. Many classic types also like pastels, but the richer ones; if they are too light or sickly you will lose your classic elegance. Traditional combinations, such as navy and white which are tiresome on others, are winners on you.

Styles Nothing extreme, but that does not mean out-of-date. Your elegance also relies on you looking current. Your proportions are balanced and you pay close attention to a good fit. The Classic Look gets lost completely if a skirt is too short or too tight, or if the jacket length is unflattering. Buy a co-ordinated look from one designer to achieve your most successful classic balance.

Make-up Your goal is an elegant polish so don't skip the complete routine of foundation, powder, blusher, eyeshadow, mascara and lipstick.

Accessories Keep it simple but never ignore the importance of earrings, your key accessory. Classic Women avoid loud, dangly, excessive styles and look best in simple, current designs, such as the large button gold/pearl earrings, the string of pearls and a quality watch.

Your shoes, like your clothes, are never extreme. The simple leather court shoe is your best bet.

Hair Never unkempt or uncontrollable, the Classic's hairstyle doesn't demand excessive daily attention; you rely on an excellent cut complementary to your face shape, with a sleek rather than a frizzy finish.

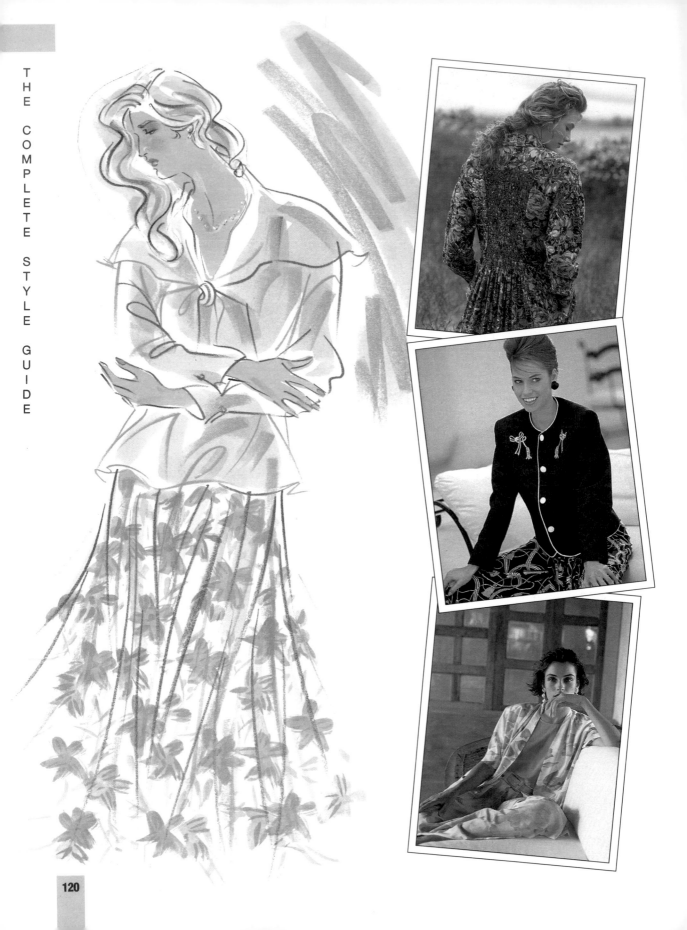

THE ROMANTIC TYPE

A TRUE Scarlette O'Hara who can create an alluring outfit from anything in your wardrobe. You are a woman who hates jeans and prefers a flowing feminine skirt and pretty blouse – even to do the gardening in.

As a Romantic Woman you pay great attention to detail, from your choice of earrings and the collar on your blouse, to the colour of your tights. You wouldn't dream of dashing out in any old thing and spend whatever time it takes (and it can take time!) to get ready.

You love colour and avoid dusty, dark shades, preferring to accent your eyes, hair and skintone with better hues (a true Color Me Beautiful convert).

Fabrics are soft, fluid and rich. Velvets, lace, silks and jersey are all favoured. Anything that begs a touch will appeal to you. Stiff suedes, tight gaberdines or anything man-made are not for the Romantic you.

Tips on Dressing Romantically

Colour   Passionate pinks, reds, plums, purples and violets worn with delicate pastel or light coloured lace and soft blouses. If you are blonde, redhead, brunette or grey you will need to adjust your colours and complement your own skintone, and eye as well as hair colour. But regardless of your Season, you will use colour in preference to neutral browns, greys, navies and black.

Styles   For work, the Romantic Woman should avoid classically tailored styles, which make you look and feel boring. Opt instead for softer cuts, which are more feminine but still professional. You will love the dress and shawl alternative to the suit as a way to express your Romantic style; just be careful not to be 'frilly' or 'silly' at the office. Off duty, blouses and skirts are your best bet.

Accessories   Your baubles are fine, delicate and detailed. Antique gold and pewter mixed with stones complement your style, along with Granny's well-worn and well-loved cameo.

Your interest in shoes can border on a fetish. With a love for detail, however, you need reminding not to go over the top and constantly reflect on the usefulness of styles. But you'll no doubt ignore advice on shoes and keep buying impulsively as a true Romantic.

Make-up   You already know that a few minutes spent on your face completes the look. Romantics do get stuck in ruts, however, so be sure you're not dating yourself by still using the same colours and techniques you applied when you left school.

Hair   No crisp cuts or functional bobs for you. If you don't have natural curls, waves or enough body to give you a sensuous style, get your hairdresser to advise. A true romantic can't be happy with sharp or limp hair.

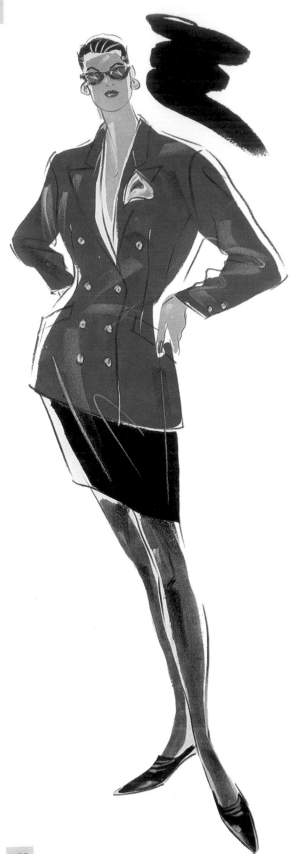

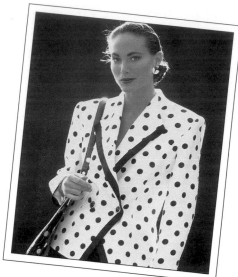

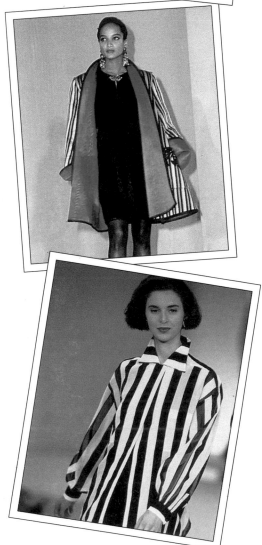

THE DRAMATIC TYPE

A BOLD, sophisticated style. You are the woman who walks into the room and knocks 'em dead with your poise, confidence and individuality.

Your colours are strong, and the primaries – red, blue and yellow – when offset against black create a favourite look. But you don't need to be a Winter Seasonal Type to achieve a dramatic effect with colour. Any woman need only choose the strongest colours from her palette and wear them in contrast.

The Dramatic Woman avoids prints, particularly anything fussy, floral or too feminine. Your choice would always be pop art, geometric or 'conversational' prints (such as a cola bottle, or smarties dancing all over your back).

Dramatics come in all shapes and sizes and don't wilt with the years (although there's great pressure to do just that). The most obvious are the tall, lean angular types who wear overscaled, striking designs so easily. Petite women with dramatic personalities can achieve the Dramatic look by avoiding obvious, cute petite clothes and choosing rather their boldest colours but in designs suited to their small scale. If you are more curved, but decidedly dramatic, let your accessories and hair create your bold, sophisticated look.

Tips for Dressing Dramatically

Colour   The primaries: reds, blues and yellows, in your Season. Solid blocks of one colour; for example, the red dress uncomplicated with anything except a simple, bold accessory. Black is a real favourite (but don't wear it close to your face if it's not in your Seasonal Palette).

Styles   Striking proportions: the long jacket and short skirt; flowing culottes with a bolero; oversized shirt with leggings. Avoid the predictable. Don't buy the complete look from one designer/manufacturer. Choose the most striking items, perhaps the jacket or skirt, to team up with something super already in your wardrobe.

Accessories   Yours have a modern edge, interpreted with sleek minimal design. Rather than lots of accessories piled on indiscriminately, select one piece as the focal point – the large brooch, striking earrings or the one-off belt. Your shoes can't be an afterthought. Go the opposite of others – the 'shoe boot' with the short skirt; the flats with trousers; the brogue with culottes.

Make-up   Your make-up must also make a statement. Best is the pale, matte foundation, deep natural tone eyeshadow (brown or grey tones) and strong lips (in your best red). Always use shades from your Seasonal Palette to achieve your dramatic look.

Hair   If straight, have it cut asymmetrically; keep short and sleek for greatest effect. If curly, an angular wedge is very dramatic. Don't forget to take your face shape into account (see page 101).

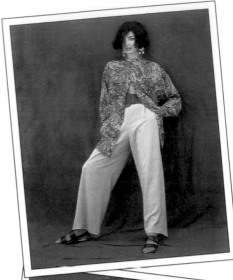

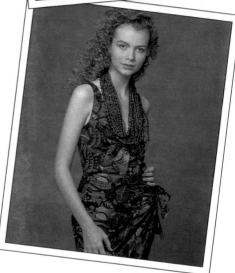

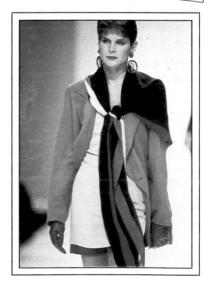

THE CREATIVE TYPE

THIS type covers the individual stylist who refuses a packaged look. If you are a younger Creative Woman you might be the body-conscious fitness freak whose wardrobe staples are your cycling shorts which you wear with sweaters and lace during the day and with sequins and stilletos at night.

The more mature Creative Type has an original look which to others is always artistic. At work, you can look professional but never stuffy because of the unpredictable way you mix separates and accessories. As a true Creative you have probably never worn the same look twice because your image always reflects your moods which, having an artistic nature, are rarely certain.

You will be expert at scouring charity shops and dress agencies for rarities passed over by others but spotted by your discerning eye.

Pressure is always there for you to be more conforming and conventional. Resist, because if you don't express your creative style you won't be able to flourish in your personal or professional pursuits.

Tips on Dressing Creatively

Colour Nothing predictable, please. Clash, astound or blend in a way no one else would dare try. Experiment with fabrics and textures that create different effects with colour, from neon Lycra to luxuriant rich velvets and tapestries. Your instinct is to shock, to amuse as well as to inspire. This is most fun for evening, weekends and on holiday. But for work don't lessen your career prospects by being deemed inappropriately dressed. At work opt for eclectic separates, using layering and accessorising to express your innovative style.

Accessories From your glasses and hair clips to your belts, buttons and boots you will want to do what isn't being done by everyone else. If you wear them, your spectacles should never be conventional neutral coloured frames. Choose a fun, bold colour instead.

Toss out belts that come with skirts and dresses and use a favoured leather one that has rich details to interpret the outfit in your own way. Hunt for unusual buttons to transform ordinary shirts and jackets.

You're the one who wears shoulder dusting earrings with great panache; never little pearl studs for the Creative Woman. Pile on beads and bangles when not working but remember to cool it for the office.

Make-up Make your eyes the focus. Define and deepen with a kohl pencil liner in a colour (never black) to enhance your eyes. For lips, start with a neutral base in your Season then accentuate the centres with your richest red.

Hair No holds barred. If your hair has good body and texture, show it off. Severe, controlled styles contradict your creative style. Take risks with colour (within your seasonal guidelines). If your hair is straight try a perm for a wild, carefree look. Just remember to control your creative tendencies for work.

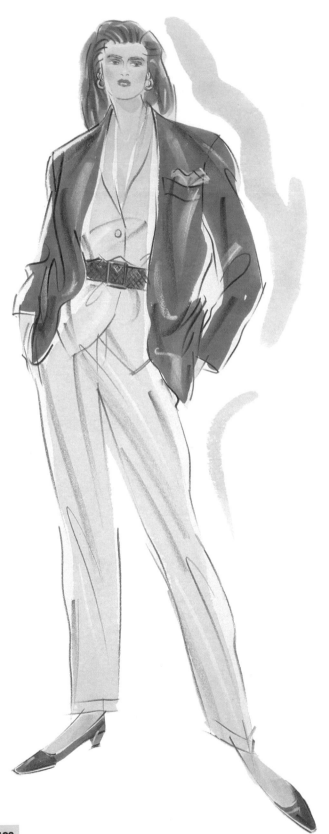

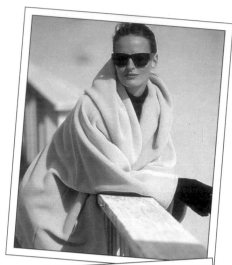

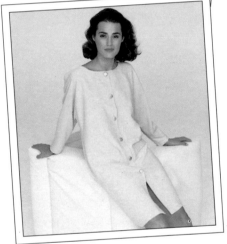

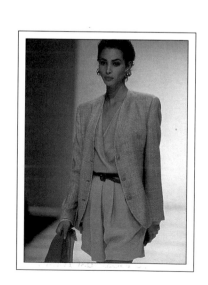

THE EUROCHIC TYPE

YOU'VE lived through many phases, perhaps as wife and mother or as a successful career woman, or as all three. After countless exhausting fashion seasons and with a wardrobe packed with too many possibilities, you eventually tired of the whole business. Today you've developed a style that has an unquestionable edge over all your contemporary fashion victims. The key to your chic is simplicity.

Your attitude is assured, elegant and relaxed. Your style reflects all that and more. In the morning you dress confident that if you were whisked off to some unknown venue or unexpected meeting you'd be well-dressed. This confidence comes from a cultivated awareness of yourself and who you are.

You might have been a Classic type in the past, but after extensive travel you realise that there are ways to look timeless and chic. You may have been a Dramatic Type who tired of uncomfortable, 'fashion-forward' styles though you still exude a very personal drama yourself.

Tips on Dressing EuroChic

Colour Blended, elegant combinations, never shades that are too bright, garish or clashing. The wardrobe staples will include ivory, charcoal, taupe, stone and pewter, which team well with monochromatic pieces or are enlivened with a dash of rich colour – olive, jade, slate or crimson. Any CMB Seasonal type can achieve the EuroChic elegance by selecting your favourite neutrals and blending them with complementary tones.

Styles Relaxed, soft and fluid, never too severe or too body hugging. An elegantly loose fit is your goal. Knits, jerseys and quality wool crêpe are terrific for cooler days, with stone-washed silks and linen for warmer ones.

Opt for good quality versus two-for-the-price-of-one bargains. The wardrobe will be lean but the possibilities will be endless.

Accessories Hunt for quality junk jewellery, avoiding extreme styles. Chanel-style costume jewellery is a good bet to complement the EuroChic look. Your accessories are important but shouldn't overpower your clothes or you.

For shoes choose updated classics and the best you can afford. For your look it's important to keep them in impeccable condition. Always tone your hosiery with your shoes for an elegant effect.

Make-up No garish or bright shades for you. Choose natural tones to complete your elegant polish and always use matte eyeshadows, never frosted or pearlised.

Hair Whether short or long, keep it in good condition. If grey is showing through be honest about its merits and if necessary get advice on options for a tint, rinse or henna treatment. Avoid frizzy perms or fussy styles.

Working *wardrobes*

WOMEN at every stage of their careers have come to us for advice on how to project a better image at work. They may want reinforcement or fine-tuning, or even a completely new look. The reasons vary but the predominant ones are:

- They were told they didn't look the part and that their appearance was adversely affecting their promotion prospects.

- They knew they were being passed over for other reasons than incompetence.

- They had let their appearance slip and didn't know how to update it.

- They had seen the transformation in a colleague and wanted similar help.

- They had overheard colleagues talking about the great image of another woman and wanted the same esteem.

Too often we've seen capable women being passed over for promotion because they didn't look or act the part. A three year study into the career progression of men and women, conducted by the Center for Creative Leadership (USA), found that out of the 100 businesses surveyed the progression of a man's career depended on competence while the progression for a woman was ability plus an acceptable image and presence. Over 35% of the woman in the study knew they had suffered criticism because of their image.

The British Institute of Manpower Studies surveyed 320 of the top UK firms in 1989 and found that more than 99% of employers still rely on the gut feeling they get about a candidate at an interview, often within minutes of setting eyes on them. The majority of recruitment in Britain is biased against women and older candidates. So if you happen to be both the cards are really stacked against you. As John Courtis explains in his book *Interviews: Skills and Strategy* there is a pervasiveness of bigotry that won't hire people who are unattractive, have 'unsuitable' hobbies or habitually wear bad shoes!

Rigorous efforts to eliminate sexual discrimination in the workplace have been slow despite comprehensive national laws and dictates from the European Commission for over 20 years. The male ranks within industry and the professions are still keeping the pace of female advancement the equivalent of a snail.

Why women hit what the Americans refer to as the 'glass ceiling' in their career advancement is the subject of much debate. Invariably the trouble starts when women are faced with the decision of whether or not to have children. Those that do automatically jeopardise their careers. They simply don't have the flexibility that their male colleagues or partners have to relocate, to travel or to work long hours when they have children. A recent survey of Britain's top 1,000 female executives found that 80% were childless. The paradox was that these same women valued health, love and *family* far above career success which scored a low 6.8%

Inadequate childcare, unreasonable work schedules and the antediluvian thinking of our macho colleagues in the male dominated boardrooms around the world will continue to affect our career prospects for a few years yet. But as more women rise to positions of power or jump ship and set up their own more flexible, enlightened and competitive businesses, the pressure should diminish. In the meantime, we'll have to accept that to get hired and climb the ladder to success we must not only have the right qualifications but look good too.

LOOKING THE PART

So what about you and your professional image. Is it working for or against you?

The right image will not only help you get promoted faster but it can also affect your earning power. A study by Clairol in 1987 involved sending two sets of CVs of talented women to prospective employers. When photos were sent with the CVs showing the candidates dressed appropriately and well-groomed, these women were offered salaries of up to 20% more than when photos showing an indifferent image were sent with identical CVs.

Another American survey (carried out by Andrew Du Brin at The Rochester Institute of Technology) found that men are more conscious of using their appearance in their career advancement than women. Thirty-five per cent of men acknowledge using their image, against 15% of women, for results on the career track. So if you aren't aware of how you need to and how you can send the right signals to get the job you want, to earn the recognition and rewards you deserve, it's time you learned. Clearly, you need to project the right image for your profession. The creative sectors (for example, advertising, marketing and the media), the fashion industry and the caring professions (such as social work and teaching) have the most choice and flexibility. More traditional professions (such as accountancy, banking, law) are still male-dominated and, hence, demand a more classic, conservative image.

So what do you do if your Style Personality (Chapter 7) is Dramatic, Romantic, Natural or Creative and you work in one of the more traditional sectors? If you really enjoy the work and are ambitious, be prepared to wear the most conservative items in your wardrobe during the day and enjoy wearing your more extreme fashions off-duty. This is not such a great compromise when you consider that one or two more 'classic' outfits earn their place in any wardrobe and quite often such clothing can be accessorised to give it more of a personalised look off-duty. Consider, too, what is at stake! I'm not 'speaking with a forked-tongue', but being practical.

Read through the Guidelines for Women Working Outside the Home and decide if you follow this advice most of the time. If not, you might be jeopardising your career prospects and possibly sending the wrong signals to your superiors, peers and subordinates.

Refer also to the specific Sector/Professions Guidelines in Chapter 9, which focus solely on the work environment or on social occasions when you mix with colleagues, clients or customers.

GUIDELINES FOR WOMEN WORKING OUTSIDE THE HOME

Styles: What to Look For

- Good quality; the best you can afford.
- Updated classics are the best investments. Use colour and accessories to create an individual look.
- Co-ordinated pieces that mix and match provide the greatest versatility. See Wardrobe Planning for your season (pages 177–180).
- Always insist on a slightly loose fit for business. Save body-conscious Lycra items for after hours (but never with clients).
- Classic not extreme skirt lengths. If your legs are an asset you can show up to 1 inch (2.5 cm) above the knee. Otherwise end your skirts at or just below the knee where the leg naturally indents.

Styles: What Not To Choose

- Inferior construction that makes the clothes look inexpensive, and you unsuccessful.
- Poor fit – too tight, too baggy, too long or too short. Any extreme in fit can make you look heavy, old and dated.
- The latest fads are bad investments for working wardrobes. Watch instead for trends: ideas and looks being used extensively that are likely to last, such as the dress and coat ensemble alternative to the suit; or the unmatched suit (that is, teamed-up separates rather than the matching suit).
- One-off designs unlikely to co-ordinate with more than one other outfit.
- Tight-fitting, bare designs. The more skin you show the less authority you'll project. This goes for the neckline, legs as well as arms (capped or short sleeves in summer are far more effective than sleeveless tops).
- The 'mini' or the maxi; the former is inappropriate and too distracting, while the latter looks dumpy and unprofessional.

Colours: What To Look For

- Begin with the neutrals from your Palette – taupe, stone, grey, navy, camel, etc. You can wear these more often without people remembering them and you can co-ordinate most of your Seasonal Palette with them to create different looks.
- Plain colours are easier to co-ordinate than patterns. Subtle weaves that blend a variety of your neutrals, such as stone, navy and ivory, are also versatile.
- The darker shades from your Seasonal Palette convey more authority than your lighter shades. But the mid-tone colours are more approachable and less threatening for days when you need to 'win friends and influence people'

Colours: What Not To Choose

- Flashy, memorable colours unless you have a basic working wardrobe of versatile neutrals. Some colours, like the reds, blues and rich greens, are striking without looking out of place, but a banana yellow or bright orange suit would look unprofessional.
- Busy, distinguishable patterns that are difficult to co-ordinate. Medium to small patterns offer greater possibilities than very bold stripes, large florals or striking checks.
- Lighter shades for suits, particularly pastels, project less authority. Save your peaches, pinks and lemon shades for blouses, scarves or in patterns. Light neutrals like taupe, stone or ivory are acceptable in business because they aren't 'ultra feminine'.

Fabrics: What To Look For *(see also the Fabric Guide on pages 181–185)*

- Natural fabrics like wool, cotton, silk, linen or blends of natural fabrics with some man-made fibres. Better to have fabrics predominantly natural, e.g. 60% wool, 40% Terylene for comfort as well as effect. The polyester suit will always look inferior to one made of wool.
- Easy-care fabrics are more practical. Check the care labels before buying.
- Matt finishes in suits, dresses, and even blouses, are more professional than shiny fabrics. Satin finishes, when used in moderation, such as a blouse under a suit, are most effective in mid-tone to deeper shades.

Fabrics: What Not To Choose

- Anything with 100% man-made fibres. Sure, they won't wrinkle, but they look tacky and cheap. Also man-made fibres don't breathe and are therefore uncomfortable to wear, particularly in the summer.
- Skimpy, sheer, fuzzy fabrics that beg to be touched. A fuzzy sweater top can never look professional whether worn alone or under a jacket.

- High maintenance fabrics, e.g. embroidered or embossed fabrics or fine silks that require dry cleaning after each wearing.
- Shiny finishes in complete outfits, such as silk, satin or leather, as you'll look dressed for the evening all day long.
- Fine cottons, linens and silks that crease so easily that you soon look shabby and unpolished.

Shoes: What to Look For

- Quality leather or suede. No plastic or fabric weaves.
- Neutral colours like black, navy or taupe are more versatile than brighter, more memorable colours.
- Same colour or slightly darker than your hemline.
- Updated classic styles in courts or pumps. Flats are very casual in look even though you may look terrific in them when wearing skirts or trousers.

Shoes: What Not To Choose

- Seasonal fashion colours that have a limited life and work with only a few items in your wardrobe.
- Stilettos or any heel that prevents you from walking normally.
- White in any style, regardless of price.

Hosiery: What To Look For

- Neutral tones to blend with your hemline.
- In winter choose 10–15 denier.
- In Summer choose 5–7 denier. Stockings and 'hold-ups' rather than tights are more comfortable in the summer.

Hosiery: What Not To Choose

- Bright colours or dramatic designs that take away from your outfit. For business your hosiery should not be making a statement but completing the polish of your look.
- Opaque, cotton or shiny Lycra.
- Going without *ever*. No matter how hot or sticky, you must wear stockings or tights for business. When commuting in summer, you could travel bare-legged but just pop into the Ladies and put on your tights before you enter the office.

Briefcase/Handbag: What To Look For

- A size that's proportionate to you. Petite women should avoid overscale large styles, while grand scale women require a bigger bag.
- A neutral colour that will co-ordinate with your suits. It doesn't need to

match your shoes, and if in a different colour it will add interest to your outfit.

- Elegant but functional in design. Consider how you like to carry your bag; if over the shoulder check the strap to see if it falls at a comfortable length. The overly functional bags with excessive zip compartments, or moulded like many inferior men's models, are unattractive for today's business women.
- One style that can accommodate both personal items and business material. Carry your make-up in a cosmetic bag and keep to a minimum of items.

Briefcase/Handbag: What Not To Choose

- Chunky, masculine styles that contradict your business image.
- Styles that are too casual or fussy and look out of place in business.
- Fashion colours that are too bright and won't co-ordinate with your whole wardrobe.
- Avoid carrying both a handbag and a briefcase as this creates a cluttered image. Find one style to accommodate everything.

GROOMING YOUR CLOTHES

Looking after your clothes is an important part of your image. Even the most expensive items will look cheap and shoddy if you don't pay attention to grooming.

Your wardrobe should only hold clothes that are ready to wear. Garments that are put away badly, are dirty or need mending will be unwearable and just clutter up the wardrobe.

Take a few minutes at the end of every day to check what needs to be done to today's outfit to ensure it's ready for another wearing. A natural bristle clothes brush is essential for brushing away dust, stray hairs and fluff. Jackets are best hung outside the wardrobe on a good, moulded hanger for at least 24 hours to breathe. Natural wool, linen, silk or cotton fibres also need air to rejuvenate them before going back into the wardrobe.

Button or zip up all fastenings before hanging things away to be sure clothes keep their shape. Use padded hangers for delicate blouses, dresses and knits and well-formed plastic or wooden hangers for jackets. Flimsy wire hangers collected with the dry cleaning do no garment justice and allow items to slip off and crease in the wardrobe. Skirts require clip-hangers or hooks for loops sewn into the inside seams.

Be sure all items are clean enough to wear again. Man-made fibres are better washed with every wearing as they retain perspiration and lose their colour and shape if left too long. It's best to launder clothes when they are only slightly dirty as heavier soil takes its wear on a garment. Always check the care label and follow the instructions for hand or machine washing or dry cleaning.

When switching your wintertime and summertime wardrobes be ruthless about cleaning. Moths and mildew are attracted to dirty, stained clothes, so ensure a longer lifetime for yours with regular care.

Dry Cleaning Tips

- For removing stains when a garment doesn't require a full cleaning, use dry cleaning fluid on a clean white handkerchief. Work from the outside of the stain inwards using small, circular rubbing motions. Keep a clean cloth, towel or handkerchief underneath the stain to absorb the excess fluid and dirt.

- Dry clean winter suits only two to three times a season. To refresh the garments hang outside on a sunny, fresh day to naturally deodorize and refresh the fibres. To remove creases, hang in a steamy bathroom or have pressed only at the dry cleaners.

- Before dry cleaning remove any shoulder pads in blouses, dresses, or jackets as they are often destroyed by the solvents.

- Remove expensive buttons if uncertain about the effects of solvents, e.g. pearl buttons lose lustre and can chip.

- Check hems and loose buttons before dry cleaning. If needing attention, ask the dry cleaner to mend (you should only use a dry cleaner that offers this service).

Shoes

Too often women treat their shoes as an afterthought when they can be the key finishing touch to an outfit. You need to aim for a few good pairs of shoes to be able to rotate them throughout the week. The 'disposable shoe' mentality (buy one pair and wear it until it falls apart then invest in another) is foolhardy; your shoes can't last if worn every day. The leather needs time to recuperate so let them rest between wearings. With care your shoes can last for years, rather than a couple of months.

Polish your shoes after wearing them as warm leather takes polish much better. Have heels and soles repaired as soon as there is any sign of wear. Often new shoes, even expensive ones, come with plastic heels which should be replaced with leather or rubber ones before wearing.

Suede shoes should be brushed with a stiff toothbrush not a wire one, even though these are often sold to care for suede (they are too sharp and damage the nap of the suede, reducing its life).

Wet shoes should never be dried near direct heat. Instead, stuff with newspaper and allow to dry in their own time, at room temperature.

Always store shoes with shoe trees in them which help them retain their shape.

Successful dressing

WE have moved from discussing how you can develop your own personal style to how to put together a wardrobe for business. Now let's consider ways of adapting your image at different stages of your career so that you always look the part and meet expectations. To be successful you must look professional.

CAREER MOVERS: THE FIRST JOB INTERVIEW

Young women entering the job market, from school, college or university, often spend an inordinate amount of time preparing their CVs but comparatively little time grooming themselves or achieving an appropriate look for the interview. You should not only look neat and tidy, but also mature and capable.

I know you're probably not flush with cash to splash out on a new wardrobe, but beg or borrow enough for a new jacket, skirt and shoes – the key elements to your business look – if your wardrobe is wanting. And read the following guidelines. They may not accord with your own ideas on 'sharp dressing' but they will help you to get and keep your first job!

A jacket – the key garment   Choose a good quality jacket in a neutral shade from your Seasonal Palette. Whether tailored or straight, it must fit well.

A skirt – keep it decent   The matching or contrasting skirt should not rise up to mid-thigh when you sit down. If you have to tug at it constantly to pull it down, it's probably too tight and too short. Just 1 inch (2.5 cm) above the knee is the limit; use a tape measure to get it right!

Smart, not silly   Avoid frilly blouses as they will either make you look younger or frivolous. Choose a smart shirt or blouse in a soft white or a light colour from your Palette that tones with your jacket and skirt.

No bare legs   Tights must be sheer, not opaque, and free of snags, holes or ladders. Take a spare pair in your handbag in case you snag them on the way to the interview.

New shoes   Choose a pair of neutral coloured court shoes; that is, with a medium heel (no flats or stilettos!).

Accessories   Keep to a minimum. Regarding earrings, button or small hoops are all that is acceptable. You're at the interview to get hired, not to get a date. Keep the style of your watch low-key; no cartoon characters on the face or fluorescent wrist straps.

Grooming essentials   Be clean and look polished. Long hair should be pulled back in a clip (no bows) or up (if you can do this efficiently).

Make-up is a must, even if you never wear it. If you have perfect skin just blusher, mascara and lipstick are minimum. If your skin isn't perfect use a light foundation to conceal blemishes. Avoid bright pearlised lipsticks or eye-shadows. See your Seasonal Palette for colour advice.

Good labels/manufacturers   Next, Marks & Spencer, Jigsaw (watch the skirt lengths), Country Casuals, Cacharel.

CAREER MOVERS: ONWARDS AND UPWARDS

Moving from entry level or dead-end jobs depends on both your abilities and your image. Assuming you've proven yourself as capable in your current position, you now need to project an image that signals to management that you are ready and able to handle greater responsibility.

To achieve recognition, among like-minded competitors, you need to stand out – to perform and look better. Here are some tips on looking right for the next career opportunity:

Dresses   Smart dresses, e.g. coat dresses, can easily be transformed into a credible business look with accessories, such as a good belt, scarves, discreet jewellery.

Jacket required   Always wear a jacket with skirts instead of a cardigan which, while sensible, looks unprofessional.

No trousers   Don't wear trousers. Senior businesswomen only wear skirts or dresses, unless running their own businesses or in more liberated environments (see pages 144–5).

Accessories   Avoid distracting accessories, like noisy earrings or bangles. Jewellery should be discreet; scarves and belts of good quality.

Be different   Do change your hairstyle if it looks like everyone else's. If long is the norm, be brave and choose a more sleek, business-like bob. If short, reshape into a more current look, depending on your face shape (see pages 101–105).

Make-up: neutral not neon   Make a real effort with your make-up. See my seven-step guide on pages 94–7. Avoid colourful eyeshadows, in favour of more neutral tones from your Seasonal Palette.

Good labels/manufacturers   Marks & Spencer, Next, Cacharel, French Connection, I Blues.

CAREER MOVERS: SWITCHING SECTORS

If planning a dramatic career switch be prepared to enter an alien business environment. They'll be wary of outsiders, expecting the negative stereotype of, for example, the typical nurse or the typical teacher. Surprise them by looking every bit the part of the new profession before you've even joined.

If coming from one of the 'caring professions', e.g. teaching, social work or nursing, into profit-orientated sectors you need to look successful. A sharp new suit says 'I'm ready for business'.

If switching from more conservative industries, like financial services, into something more creative, e.g. consumer products, you'll need to jazz-up your act. Check your Seasonal Colour Palette for more interesting colour combinations than those you normally wear. Make sure your accessories are current; most women working in conservative sectors – insurance, banking, accounting – tend to wear accessories that are five or more years out-of-date.

In researching a career move – even before an interview – try to get an idea not only about career prospects, but also about the business culture. Visit the office building and observe people coming and going through the foyer or front entrance. How fashionably are they dressed? How safe do they play it? Also study the chart on pages 144–5.

Study the company brochure for key words describing the corporate identity. If 'reliable', 'trustworthy' and 'professional' are much used, for example, you can be sure that they will want their staff to look so as well. So in this instance wear a classically tailored suit, looking current, but on the conservative side.

Forget what you own   Assume that some – or most – of your wardrobe is not appropriate for your new career and be prepared to invest in a top-to-toe new look; a new suit, appropriate earrings, and shoes. See the Guidelines for building a Basic Working Wardrobe on pages 148–150.

Sell yourself   Look approachable. The colours you choose can help you present an image to potential employers that says you are willing to listen to *their* needs. Navy suits and white blouses make the sell harder. Instead, choose mid-tone colours offset with a bright blouse to make you look more approachable.

Good labels/manufacturers   Paul Costello, Jaegar, Mondi, Marella, Windsmoor, Max Mara.

CAREER MOVERS: UP TO MANAGEMENT

Often women stuck in career ruts have created their own terminal conditions by dressing and behaving inconsistently and unlike a manager. Unfortunately, this is not the place to give guidance on how to be more assertive, on achieving more involvement in management activities that make your promotion certain, on how to build a small team that requires your leadership and wins inevitable recognition. Suffice it to say that, in addition to some shrewd manoeuvring, you also need to look like a manager.

Are there any role models in your organisation, women in management, from whom you could learn a few pointers in dressing successfully? Do they consistently look the part? If so, you need to as well. If you occasionally shock management by wearing silly, inappropriate clothes they are unlikely to appoint you to their team and risk you turning up badly dressed for a client meeting or in any situation, planned or ad hoc, when you would be representing the company.

Time to upgrade   A promotion requires a good quality image; you need to look the part even before you get there. Learn to recognise good quality and proper fit and be prepared to pay for both.

Investment priorities   Be prepared to spend at least four weeks' take-home salary on your business wardrobe every year to maintain your successful image.

Go neutral   Switch from bright and pastel colours to quality neutral tones which project more authority. Check your Seasonal Colour Palette for tips on your best neutral choices. Wear in solids or weaves, blending a few tones together. Use your favourite brights and pastels as accents, i.e. in scarves, blouses, pocket hankies.

Accessories give the edge   Invest in the best your budget allows including: quality leather shoes, religiously polished and re-heeled; three smart pairs of quality 'fake' earrings (try Monet, Napier, Ken Lane); at least two good leather belts to complete your suits; a beautiful shawl-sized scarf to brighten up coats and jackets.

Good labels/manufacturers   Austin Reed, Paul Costello, Mani, Jaegar, Harvey Nichols (own label), Marella, Nichol Fahri, J.H. Collectibles.

CAREER MOVERS: ON TO THE BOARD

The boardrooms of companies around the world accommodate far too few female directors at a time when women's talents are needed, more than ever, in all types of industry and every profession. For many women, the elevator of success stops just below the boardroom suite. They can see through the 'glass ceiling' but somehow are prevented from reaching the top, often because of their image.

There's little point in getting mad about the situation. You've just got to persist in showing by every means you have that you can meet the challenge as well as – and better than – the next man. Tough – yes – but not impossible. More and more women *are* making the breakthrough and so can you.

So the challenge is mind reading. Women are so much more intuitive than men – this is easier than it sounds. If you are the first woman to be up for appointment you'll need a look similar in tone and quality to the men. If some wear jazzy ties and colourful shirts you can have some fun yourself. If they are a sober pinstripe and white shirt brigade you'll need to look sober yourself.

I can't help you get the right qualifications and experience; that's something you'll have to work at. But I certainly can help you to look destined for the board – and even, in the fullness of time, its head. Let's make a start.

Suits safest   Unless in creative sectors, dresses are a risk when you're aiming for the top. Smart suits, preferably with matching rather than contrasting skirts, are best.

Get the real thing   Fakes may have been fine until now but, for the boardroom, 'real' accessories are required. A good watch, quality earrings, brooches and chokers are what you need to smarten up your sober suits.

If you show too much you'll blow your chances   For corporate events held in the evening choose appropriate styles: elegant but understated – you're still working. Many women destroy their corporate chances by not knowing how to dress outside the office; the more skin you show the more power you lose.

Stylish signature   For meetings, use a leather file for transporting papers and a quality fountain pen to take notes. Disposable biros and felt tips are fine for making drafts back at your office, but not in meetings with colleagues or the board.

Smell special   Use a light fresh scent daily, avoiding anything too heady; you don't want the scent to arrive before you and hang around long after you've made your mark and left. Avoid perfume; choose cologne or eau de toilette instead.

Keep your head   Have an attractive, not 'butch' hairstyle. Busy business women with little time to spend on grooming their hair too often opt for sensible but too severely cropped styles which can be very unattractive. Potential board partners don't want a male clone, they want a female partner. So hair, make-up, accessories and clothes, while appropriately restrained, should always be feminine.

Make-up   Spend at least 10 minutes on it in the morning and touch up your lipstick and powder throughout the day every time you visit the cloakroom.

Professional help   Research nearby services for hairdressing, facials and beauty treatments, and dental treatment and book them into your diary regularly.

Good labels/manufacturers   Donna Karan, Armani, Valentino, Chanel, Krizia, Jill Sander, Gignetti, Cerutti.

CAREER MOVERS: WOMEN RETURNERS

There's no such thing as a non-working woman; there are just some who don't get paid. And now it's time for you to get paid for your talents. Maybe the children have grown up or your partner has learned how to cope without a 24 hour attendant. Just a few low hurdles to clear and you'll be back in the mainstream. Here's how.

Mid-career, middle-aged women returners often signal under-confidence and look like someone's mum the minute they walk through the door. That's two marks against you. If your CV can't boast some previous job experience it's three marks! Don't despair. Your body language can say the right things for you at an interview if you follow the advice in Chapter 11, and your clothes and make-up can boost a good first impression even more. Also your CV can be drafted to translate all those years in 'Home Management' into relevant, employable experience.

The key is not to look dated, but to look timeless. Brace yourself to be interviewed by someone 10–20 years your junior, who isn't hiring a mother figure but a co-worker. You need to do some preliminary investigation yourself and find out how everyone else dresses at that particular organisation *before* the interview; afterwards is too late.

The good news is that it is slowly becoming chic to be middle-aged, because more of us are so. By the year 2000, 35–44 year olds will dominate the population; by the year 2015 most of us will be over 45. So you don't need to look 'young' although you don't need to age yourself unnecessarily with a lethargic expression, a dated hairstyle or middle-aged spread. 'Positive and current' is what you want to signal.

Here are the tips which I dole out with brutal honesty to help returners like you to get the jobs you seek:

Smart dressing   The floral Laura Ashley dress you simply love won't impress at a job interview, even when teamed with a smart jacket. A good up-to-date jacket with a matching or contrasting skirt is what is required. Buy the best quality you can afford for instant appeal and lasting effect.

In good trim   If you haven't made up your mind whether you like or hate your grey hair, it's decision time. Unless it's a gorgeous shade and suits you well, eliminate it with a rinse in a shade lighter than your natural colour – but have it done professionally. And while you're in the chair, why not decide on an up-to-date and flattering new style? You'll lose 10 years immediately.

Smart trappings   Good accessories will complement your new outfit and set you above other anxious returners in the interview queue. Think of any necessary expenditure as an investment that will pay off.

Saving face   Many returners appreciate that make-up is important for an interview. The only problem is that they are applying theirs the same way they did 10 or 20 years ago. Learn some new tricks. Update your make-up to help you look fresh, healthy and professionally polished. See also pages 94–7.

On the right scent   If your budget will take the strain, do wear a classy light fresh scent to further enhance your chances

Good labels/manufacturers   Marks & Spencer, Paul Costello, Jaegar, Marella, Betty Barclay.

CAREER MOVERS: INTO PUBLIC LIFE

As someone who started her career in politics, I'm an advocate of more women holding public office. National politics remains essentially a male domain although strides are being made in many countries with elected chambers organising their business to accommodate the pressures on working wives and mothers.

Increasingly women are attracted to seeking elected positions whether it be the local school board, city council or as a national representative. To be chosen through the democratic voting process you need to be convincing on the issues and look the part to convince the electorate that you can do the job.

Television has changed the demands on all politicians. Whether they like it or not they have to look well-groomed, not just to compete against their opponents, but to overcome voter apathy and make people select *them* as their representative. See pages 147–8 for advice on appearing on television.

Once in the political ring it's too late for a new (or improved) image; if you change too much when campaigning your image becomes a campaign issue. Take note of the following tips for a winning public image.

Before you hit the trail   If unsure, make an appointment with an image consultant to find out exactly what colours, styles and make-up will suit you, and get them to plan your campaign wardrobe. A little planning beforehand will help you focus your energies on the issues, not worry about what you are going to wear tonight. See Working Wardrobe options listed at the end of this chapter.

Rotate your shoes   Because of the demanding foot work on the campaign trail, you will be tempted to wear sensible but often unflattering shoes. Instead, choose several alternative pairs with low heels (more flattering with a suit) and rotate them throughout the day, changing up to three times if needed to revitalise the feet.

Look approachable   Dreary, dark shades can put off voters or supporters. Check your Seasonal Palette for brighter, more winning colours (also see Your Colour Vitamins, Chapter 4) to help you suceed in looking approachable, capable and interesting.

Trousers OK   When campaigning, and if your figure allows, a smart trouser suit can work as well as a dress or skirt. It can also be much more practical when working in rural areas. But always change to a suit to give a speech. For rural constituents be sure you don't overwhelm them in a slick, 'power suit'. Opt instead for tweed, houndstooth or other less fussy, 'country' fabrics.

Not a hair out of place   Assume there is a camera around every corner, so your hairstyle needs to be neat and manageable as well as attractive. Also no roots showing. Have non-aerosol hairspray available at all times as well as a comb and mirror for necessary touch-ups. If your hair is difficult to manage, get a better cut and/or perm to make upkeep easier.

Once elected stand out   On days you plan to make a statement wear colours that will help you stand out in the crowd. Very bright colours like red or fuchsia will bleed on camera (i.e. go fuzzy) and be too distracting once you begin speaking. Wear a bright blouse under a neutral suit rather than a whole suit in banana yellow for best effect.

Avoid twinky touches   Fussy bows and scarves, distracting jewellery and useless handbags all take away from your stature as a woman MP, councillor or senator. Smart, contemporary earrings or choker, simple gold chain and/or pearls are best. Never appear without your earrings, they are the equivalent in importance for a woman as a tie is for a man.

Good labels/manufacturers   The best of your own national designers/ manufacturers.

CAREER MOVERS: FROM PARTNER TO EXECUTIVE WIFE

Corporate entertaining is all about public relations, creating good feelings within a company and with their customers. Many wives have to face up to the responsibility of being a hostess or guest at formal dinners, cocktail parties and special events like conferences abroad, the races, sailing, shooting or skiing weekends. Some women thrive in the role while others consider it a chore and a tedious waste of time. But remember, how you perform as an Executive Wife can affect the progress of your husband's career and the financial rewards for you and your family. So there's a vested interest in you succeeding in the role.

Teamwork   You and your husband are a team so your image should mirror his, that is, the company's expectations of him. If he's a dynamic, 'up and coming' star you need to project a promising image as well. If you are shy and reserved you can look otherwise by dressing more dramatically. By looking like a team I don't mean matching outfits, just complementary images.

Boss's wife sets the style   If it's your first event, find out what the boss's wife is like and how she usually dresses for such occasions. If your husband has attended other such occasions but is a bit vague on details, personal assistants or secretaries can be very helpful – but do be discreet in your enquiries.

Play safe   Don't risk the all-important first impression by over-dressing or looking too seductive. If you are attractive, fit and young don't flaunt it as an Executive Wife – other wives will resent it if you receive excessive attention.

Fake it 'til you make it   Positive body language and a confident voice are essential to the Executive Wife. When entering a room full of unfamiliar faces, stride in confidently, quick paced as if you can't wait to meet everyone. Use direct eye contact. Repeat everyone's name when introduced: 'Marilyn, lovely to meet you': 'Hello George'. Smile often (but not when inappropriate!). And train your husband to thank you for every performance.

COMBINING PERSONALITY AND PROFESSIONAL IMAGE

Today women realise that they need to consider the occasion, the audience and the sector or industry when they are putting together their look or developing an image to help them get ahead.

The chart on the following pages provides a quick reference for various industries concerning options for daytime styles, use of colour, accessorising, and business entertainment. These guidelines stem from extensive experience working within different sectors, as well as observation of what works and should stand you in good stead if in doubt about how to dress for clients or occasions. Once you read the guidelines it's up to you, at this stage of your career, to decide to what extent it is advisable to follow them and play it safe.

Remember that these are just guidelines – above all it's important to feel confident and comfortable. Let your common sense guide you on what is right for *you* while at the same time being appropriate for the occasion. And don't forget those Colour Vitamins (Chapter 4).

Sector/Professions	Daytime Style Options	Use of Colour
'Serious' Professions e.g. law, banking, accounting, insurance	Limited: suits only. Updated classics best. No flimsy fabrics, high heels, nor elaborate accessories.	Limited: understatement is the goal. Blend tones of one colour or wear a bright blouse to enliven sober suits.
Professional 'People-Orientated' Sectors e.g. management consulting training, marketing, P.R.	For client meetings suits only but mix 'n' match jackets with skirts. Dresses are fine for the office. No trousers unless Fashion P.R.	Wear power colours like red for presentations, mid-tone neutrals for client meetings.
Sales – High Tech e.g. computer software, engineering products, medical supplies	A professional look needed: suits only. Classics with flair.	Avoid navy and white. Try mid-tone neutrals with blouses in soft pastels for a more 'user-friendly' look.
Sales – Consumer Products and Services e.g. estate agents, hotel and catering	Professional yet more fashionable look than your high-tech counterparts. Choose suits with current proportions, not too classic.	Go for the red jacket with grey tweed skirt and you will get noticed.
Direct Selling e.g. double-glazing, cosmetics and fashion products, slimming instructors	Consider your clients and choose quality and style that might inspire them (not over the top just aspirational – 'I could look like that'), and that instil confidence.	If your product is serious, opt for blended neutrals. If fashion or beauty, look colourful.
Creative e.g. advertising, retail, media, publishing, travel	Fashionable suits are best. Smart trouser suits are a viable alternative if good quality and they suit you.	Abandon the clone-colours and black if in this sector. Use your Palette creatively.
Caring Sectors e.g. social services, medical (non-uniformed), counsellors	Co-ordinates that mix and match are most practical. Make-up is essential to look fresh when you're exhausted.	High contrast shades that aren't threatening, e.g. navy with white. Use colour to cheer up as well as win confidence of patients.
Teaching e.g. schools, colleges	Make the effort. Be inspirational. Attempt to look current but not funky.	Don't play too safe and sensible. Surprise occasionally. Interesting colours to hold but not distract pupils' attention.

Accessories	Dinner After Hours 'Still on Duty'	Evening: Formal with Colleagues/Clients
A good watch, classic but current earrings, two rings maximum, end of discussion.	Wool crêpe makes a good transition day to night. Strengthen make-up, change blouse to a silk or satin one.	No décolletage or strapless styles. Stunning not sexy.
More flair allowed than Serious Professions (above) but nothing wayout. Current classics are best.	Opt for more colour and different accessories for evening.	See 'Serious' Professions.
Keep them as an afterthought, never obvious. But don't go without.	Keep the look professional, especially if still selling. Change blouse to a silk or satin one.	No dreary black. Be colourful and fun but not risqué.
Current but professional. No distracting baubles.	Colourful flair required. Dresses fine provided not too frilly or too slinky.	Chic and charming. Strapless only if you are hostess (you set the tone) not the guest (it might offend).
Excessive beads, bangles and baubles are out of place in the home sales environment.	Less pressure if selling to other women. If mixed company be chic and discreet.	Have fun, express your personality. If your tendency is to go too far e.g. with make-up, accessories or revealing décolletage, pull back: soften the make-up and eliminate one accessory.
Current, that make a statement. But tone-down if working with cautious, conservative clients.	Keep it professional but fashionable. Your hairstyle is the key to your look. Add discreet hair accessories.	Don't go overboard or you'll lose authority. See Sales – Consumer Products and Services.
A nice pair of earrings is all that's necessary.	Make the time to do a minor transformation. Change shoes from flats to moderate heels. Add some sparkle in earrings or in a brooch.	You want to surprise and startle. No dreary shades. Let your personality come through. Opt for prints rather than solid fabrics.
Too much will distract pupils. Earrings will command respect.	Dresses and trouser suits are fine.	You are still a role model so beware of looking too flash or seductive; you might worry others about your influence on pupils.

YOUR PRESENTATION IMAGE

I'm often asked for advice on what to wear when giving a presentation. To be most helpful, I need to know the purpose of the meeting, the objectives to be achieved and the anticipated size of the audience. But I can give you some useful advice that applies to public speaking in general.

Any presentation demands a strong, complementary visual image. You have to expect your audience to drift off from time to time during your talk. To bring their attention back you need to vary the pace of your delivery and use visual aids – of which *you* are the most important one.

You can learn a great deal from observing others, so become a critic at every presentation you attend. Take notes of what you felt was strong about the presenter's image and what you felt let her/him down. Learn from your own mistakes as well: ask for constructive criticism after each of your presentations. Find out what people liked, what they learned and remembered and how your image and presence came across.

The Business Presentation

The smaller the audience the softer, less threatening your look should be. A boardroom presentation to a group of 10 doesn't require the snappy red suit. In situations where you are close to your audience you want to use colour in moderation – too much can overwhelm. Go for neutral coloured suits and introduce more colour with your blouse. If you concentrate the colour near your face it will work like a spotlight focussing attention on you and what you are saying.

The large audience presentation becomes 'theatre' and therefore requires a 'costume'. The navy-suited speaker at a conference of 500 people is unlikely to make much impact or hold the audience's attention. This is the occasion to bring colour into your jacket, if not your whole suit. Try the brighter colours from your Palette – which should still be appropriate for business – to win audience attention. Note that any boldness should be from plain colours and subtle fabrics, never large patterns which are too distracting.

Check the lighting in the room before any presentation. You may work in modern conference centres with perfectly regulated lighting as well as dimly lit theatres and exhibition halls. If the dais from where you'll be speaking is dark, you'll need to 'brighten it up' by wearing lighter, brighter shades.

Style Tips

When selecting styles consider how your body reacts under the stress of giving a presentation. If you're the type who needs to move, to gesture to release the adrenalin pumping through your body, then be sure your clothes allow plenty of movement. Avoid strict, straight skirts or tight jackets. Always keep your jacket buttoned when speaking so there are no distractions (e.g. your bosom, waist or tummy). Avoid high heels; when you are nervous you want to have all the confidence possible – without worrying about tripping or falling.

TIPS FOR APPEARING ON TELEVISION

The prospect of appearing on television can be very daunting. The newsreaders with whom we are so familiar make it look very easy when in reality it is not. If we watch news interviews or panel discussions with amateurs (much like ourselves), we know how badly people can come across and how their appearance can let them down. It's very difficult to listen to someone who is wearing bright lipstick, a loud scarf, a flashy necklace, or whose hair is too fussy. All we do is watch the lips, the clothes, or the hair and are too distracted to actually listen to what is being said.

For the past few years I've worked in conjunction with media trainers in coaching individuals to handle interviews. We help them develop the content of their message and work on projecting the right image through their appearance, expressions and voice.

Here are some basic tips on dressing for television, whether you are a professional presenter or an amateur interviewee.

Clothing

- The key is to wear simple outfits without any fuss to distract from your face.
- Wear colours from your Palette from the middle of the colour spectrum (blues, greens, purple) which aren't too light, dark or bright. Avoid red which tends to 'bleed' on camera, i.e. the edges run and look fuzzy.
- A monochromatic blend of colours (suit and blouse of different shades of one colour) is best. Avoid sharp contrast, e.g. black and white or bold prints. Stripes, herringbones and plaids can 'dance' or 'move around' on screen.
- Avoid plunging necklines.

Jewellery

- Avoid dangling earrings which will distract viewers' attention.
- Less is best. Gold and pearl combinations look most elegant.
- If wearing large earrings don't wear a necklace as well. Instead balance with a simple brooch.
- Don't wear noisy bangles or clanking chains. The viewers want to hear you – not your jewellery.
- Don't wear any jewellery with smooth shiny surfaces which could cause problems with reflections.

Make-up

- Most studio lighting is very harsh on the skin and penetrates three layers, so make-up is essential.
- Always wear foundation, and a heavier type than normal. Choose a colour to match your skintone or darker.
- It's important to use concealer to balance any dark areas, particularly around the eyes; television lighting will emphasise them.
- For eye make-up a peach-base shadow with a grey contour is best. Browns make your eye look bruised; blues and other such colours appear too harsh and distracting on camera.

- Use blusher to contour your face (otherwise it will look flat). Use matt powder only.
- Choose natural shades of lipstick. Avoid reds, pale and bright pinks or dark browns and burgundies, and anything too bright or distracting.
- Powder your face heavily to avoid any shine.
- Easy does it with the mascara. Natural colours – black, brown or grey – only.

Hairstyle

- Your hair is there to frame your face. Keep it simple and not distracting. Clip, tie or spray hair if it's likely to fall across your face.
- Make sure the cut and volume compliment your face (see Chapter 6).
- If you colour your hair, be sure it's always done before a TV appearance. Tell-tale roots are always ghastly but particularly so on television.

Glasses

- Glasses create a barrier between you and the viewer, so avoid wearing them if possible. Otherwise get a pair with non-reflective lenses.
- Never wear tinted glasses on camera.

THE BASIC WORKING WARDROBE

For women starting out, returning to work or wanting to completely overhaul their working wardrobes and begin afresh, below I suggest a capsule collection of items which will provide the foundation for building a terrific wardrobe. See also the advice for Career Movers on pages 135–143, and Wardrobe Planning for Your Season on pages 177–180.

Select a Colour Scheme

Refer to your Seasonal Colour Palette and see what colours I have put together for the business outfit. If you like them, you can plan your basic working wardrobe around those colours. If not, don't worry, simply select other neutrals and colours from your Palette to team together.

Opt for High Quality

Since this will be your foundation wardrobe, choose the best quality you can afford; your investment priorities should be suits and shoes.

Suits

Your goal will be to have two suits that can be interchanged to create different looks. The first investment should be a terrific jacket in a deep neutral, such as olive, charcoal or navy; the second jacket can be a lighter neutral, such as stone, pewter or medium grey. Collarless jackets will give you more flexibility with different blouses to wear underneath. For style, select current or classic looks that suit your figure. Medium weight fabrics such as wool crêpe, botany wool and light gabardine will be most versatile for up to 10 months of the year. If your climate is warmer, buy one suit in a lighter weight – cool wool or a cotton blend.

Knitted Top and Skirt

If knits compliment your figure, select a matching top and skirt that can be worn together or separately. Opt for generous, not body-hugging designs in rich, mid-tone shades to work with your neutral jackets and skirts depending on your Palette, perhaps terracotta with aubergine; periwinkle blue with grey; or raspberry with taupe.

Printed Two-Piece or Dress

Choose a fabric, pattern and style that teams well with your suits. The colours can be brighter to liven up your neutral basics. Aim for maximum mix-and-match potential.

Blouses

Buy three blouses in plain colours from your Seasonal Palette: choose your best white, red, and pastel.

For interest, look for blouses with attractive buttons (or replace indifferent ones) and in fabrics with a 'self-pattern'; for example, a satin stripe or simple design in the fabric. Best in quality cotton, silk, or a natural blend.

Trousers

If your figure and profession make trousers an option, choose a good quality gabardine pair in a neutral colour, to tone with your jackets.

Coat Dress

A simple, wool crêpe coat dress looks elegant on its own or can be transformed with accessories. For example, you can add a good belt or colourful scarf, or wear it with a suit jacket. This dress can take you from day to evening if you add accessories such as gold and pearl chains, or an interesting brooch. Choose a favourite colour from your Palette that can also work with the suit jacket if worn. Purple, red or turquoise are good choices.

Three-piece Evening Ensemble

Don't wait for that unexpected dinner invitation, but look now for that something special for evening that will be elegant as well as versatile, and that will last you for a few years. It's best to go for an outfit in mid-tone to deep shades (e.g. bronze, purple, navy) in silk, satin or fine wool crêpe. The three pieces would be:

- A simple unstructured jacket, which you can also wear – buttoned-up with a toning skirt or unbuttoned over a slimline dress – to the office
- A camisole or T-shirt, which will be handy for transforming your suits convincingly into after-six looks
- A long skirt or trousers; you can eventually add another printed top to go with these.

Overcoat

Decide if a mackintosh or a wool coat is a better bet for your climate. Make sure it's ample enough in cut to wear over suits. Long, mid-calf lengths are most flexible as they stay wearable however much skirt lengths vary. But petite women should choose to just below the knee length designs (provided they don't wear longer skirts).

Shoes

If you work full-time you need at least three pairs. Start with two pairs of medium heels and one with a low-to-stacked heel which will be fine with trousers. Flat shoes are very limiting unless you are very tall. Suede or plain leather styles with minimal features are the most versatile. Choose from your best neutral colours – black, brown, navy, olive, mahogany or burgundy.

Scarves

Medium-sized silk squares or long scarves can liven-up your neutral basics. If you like wearing scarves, learn several tying tricks to enable you to wear yours differently every time. Long ones can be used as sashes, too, if you are trim.

A large, colourful shawl in fine wool can serve to brighten up your coat or a plain dress if worn as a 'jacket' (tied over your shoulders) in the evening. Beware though if you have a very short neck; the shawl will ride up round your chin – warming but not very flattering – and will emphasise your shortcoming.

Belts

Choose quality leather or suede belts to wear with skirts or trousers and to accent your dress. A belt completes the look of a skirt and helps to anchor a blouse if it is worn tucked in, but make sure it is the right shape and width for your figure type. Choose the same colours as your shoes.

Shoulder Bag/Briefcase

A large, envelope style shoulder bag can double up as handbag and briefcase. If you need a more professional look invest in a good briefcase or document case, but never use it in addition to a handbag.

Jewellery

The essentials include:

- A good watch in a simple style and modest size.
- Two pairs of earrings – gold, gold and pearl, or gold and silver – in updated classic styles.
- A brooch; not necessarily to match earrings but to add interest to jackets.
- A gold chain to enhance blouses and add interest in the evening.

Hosiery

Non-shiny, Lycra blends give the best fit and are successful on different shaped legs. Avoid very dark, opaque tights and stockings or ones with textured patterns. Tone to blend with your shoes and/or your hemline.

chapter ten

Cross cultural image

COLOR Me Beautiful's network spans over 35 countries and consists of a diverse multi-cultural team. Every year we meet at our annual convention in London and, despite the cultural differences, the unique markets, and specialised national approaches, we learn a great deal from each other. We are all concerned with helping our clients make the most of themselves, and we employ the same basic techniques I have already shared with you in this book. However, the approaches used by each consultant vary in response to the unique interests and traits of their particular cultures.

Leading up to 1992 in Europe focussed attention on the inevitable globalisation of trade and the impact, too, of a worldwide, interrelated economy. In fact, global fashion has already been with us for well over a decade. In Milan young teenagers are sporting American 501 Levis and James Dean T-shirts. In Britain, working women are favouring the international professional ease typified by the Americans, Donna Karan and Calvin Klein – but provided by other astute manufacturers at more affordable prices. In California, elegant hostesses prefer the European chic of Versace, Ungaro and Armani over flashy native designs. Young and middle-aged Russians alike are still willing to forego a month's salary for Western jeans and baseball caps, and English logo sweatshirts.

But even though the opportunities to share fashion across national boundaries have increased, it doesn't mean that we'll soon all be dressing alike. Working women around the world universally aim for a professional, stylish image, whether they're living in Sydney, Chicago or Frankfurt, but they tend to adapt current styles in keeping with their national culture. Americans have had a perpetual love affair with English country style typified by the designer Ralph Lauren. But you always can tell when it's an American underneath the English-style garb. You'd never see a native Brit in a Laura Ashley dress teamed with Reeboks, a lacquered hairstyle and 2 inch red fingernails, for example.

Frequently reactions to the way women of different nationalities dress are condescending, 'How typically American/German/Australian'. Rather than be judgemental and stereotype the millions of women we have worked with, I want to share with you aspects of their image that are important to them, so that we might all learn for each other as well as be more readily accepted when we visit their country.

When travelling abroad, language is the first important hurdle. Just a smattering of everyday courtesies and greetings will win appreciation from the host citizens, so do spend time beforehand learning a few basic phrases.

If you are planning a trip, especially on business, you'll also want to know ahead of time what style will be most appropriate for the occasions planned, and what image will be most acceptable to your host/client. Space here allows for me to give only cursory insights for a few selected countries on the importance of image and what you need to consider before a visit, but in the Bibliography you will find recommendations for further reading, if this subject is of particular interest to you.

FRANCE

Here is a country where style matters at every level, from the uniformed Parisian police force to students and business executives. The French have what the Americans might call an 'attitude' problem. They can be deprecating about other nationalities' sense of style because they believe that design and good taste are the purview of the French – it's in their genes. Once you accept this, you'll get along fine when visiting France or meeting French visitors in your country.

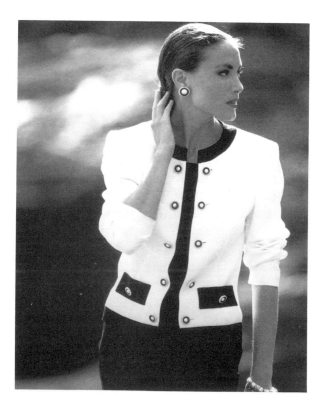

French chic

Putting national pride aside, there's a lot to be learned from their appreciation of style, which they cultivated as children at *maman*'s knee. Here are a couple of useful pointers.

Hair Whiling away the time in a Parisian café you will be struck by the smart hairstyles of most French women. Their hair looks healthy and perfectly groomed but rarely contrived. The French aren't impressed by the latest asymmetrical look but prefer timeless, yet current chic.

Many visit the hairdresser on a weekly basis. In most places, salons are open late in the evenings, as well as on Sunday mornings to accommodate this national passion for perfectly groomed hair. A shoulder length bob is preferred by many French women since this is easily adapted for different looks for the office, evening or when just relaxing at weekends.

One Outfit, a Hundred Possibilities The French woman values quality over quantity. Unlike Americans who love to have a back-up of possible options packed into their wardrobe, the French believe less is best. They are very astute planners, and will preview the season's offerings before deciding which outfit they simply can't live without.

Once purchased, the season's outfit is displayed regularly. Other nationalities may go to great lengths not to be seen wearing the same thing within a week, but the French are proud to display the special outfit time and again, not only because they know it always looks terrific and is current, but because each time 'the outfit' is worn it takes on a new guise. The shoes may be switched from heels to little suede boots, to flats. On one occasion the suit is sober and simple, then next time it is worn with a bright clashing scarf. The jacket may be belted one day then unbelted the next. It will be teamed up with other choice items from last year, perhaps dressed up with a chiffon skirt or played down with Lycra leggings.

Travel Tips

In business, expect a lot of formality. The French are great joiners of associations and committees and decorate their letterheads and signatures with lots of distinctions. Handshaking is brisk and always done with alacrity upon meeting. A positive *'bonjour'* when entering a taxi, shop or restaurant is expected; should you forget you'll be dismissed as a 'peasant'.

When visiting France your clothes don't need to be expensive or French to be successful. The only caveat is to look current. Get the proportions right first and foremost. If 'current' is a long $7/8$ jacket with a shorter skirt, try to create this look within your own wardrobe. If in doubt, play it simple with smart, knitted separates, such as a long cardigan, culottes and top or a beautiful knitted dress (just get the length right). What makes the French wince is anything that looks dated.

Pay close attention to your grooming, too. Particular care is needed for your nails, hair and make-up. No false, New York-style nails are required, just perfectly manicured and well-buffed tips. If your hair styling techniques are a bit tired, treat yourself to an update by a local hairdresser before an important meeting or social event. On the subject of make-up, nothing ornate is necessary, but never be without. I'm talking about attention to detail uncommon in Germany, the UK, America, Scandinavia – anywhere! In France even the men notice when you've had your hair done, they appreciate the colour as well as the quality of your hosiery, and can even recognise your perfume by name. When the men are this attentive you can imagine the scrutiny you will be under from the women!

GERMANY

The German lifestyle can best be described as controlled and conservative. In this regulated society, there are rules for everything – from what you plant in your garden to when you can and cannot wash your car or sweep your path to forbidding you to play the piano at lunchtime if you live in an apartment block. Germany's conservatism in the last decades has been the reason for its success.

One of the dominant values in Germany is ecology. The German Greens did more to establish the environmental movement in Europe than any other nationality. Today it is less tyrannical, less utopian than it was a decade ago, but it is still a very important issue. Like the French, German women are not impulsive shoppers; they have wholeheartedly accepted the precept that more is wasteful and less is best. Because of their ecological concerns and penchant for quality, they proudly wear a few outfits every season rather than parade a new look every day.

Unlike the British, who defy conformity, the Germans praise it in the spirit of egalitarianism: Germany is successful, therefore all Germans deserve to look good. They spurn conspicuous consumption and ostentatious displays of wealth.

The fashions distinguish themselves not by innovation or design but by quality. In every price range you'll find well-made clothes which are also increasingly found in mass market shops throughout Europe. However, the names on their labels are anything but German sounding: Betty Barclay, Escada, Mondi, I Blues.

Rarely are there major swings in fashion. Fluctuating hemlines which cause concern in other countries are dismissed as trivial by this nation of sensible women, more bent on value for money than being currently chic.

Travel Tips

German women are taller and bigger-boned than many other Western Europeans. Therefore, they prefer loose, unstructured, easy designs to body-hugging or fussy styles. In business, opt for a more formal suit in keeping with the more formal way in which meetings are conducted.

Over a business lunch expect important matters to be dealt with immediately, after ordering. This is in complete contrast to the French who consider it barbaric to mix business discussion with dining.

But the strict formality in business is often greatly contrasted when you meet with Germans socially. If invited to their homes you'll be more warmly welcomed than anywhere else.

Keep the glitz to a minimum for evening; diamanté, sequins and glitter are considered tacky. Layered silk ensembles (see page 149) are your best bet for 'after six'. Like the Swedes, the Germans mix textures beautifully – knits with suede, satin-trimmed leather; hand-knitted, hand-painted fabrics. But before you do any shopping here yourself, check the strength of the D-Mark, otherwise you could be in for a real shock. Bargains in Germany are few and far between.

ITALY

When I asked my European consultants which women, in their opinion, had the most natural style, the Italians were first choice. They achieve their reputation without the fastidiousness of the French but with a passion for design – and by always looking their best. Even popping out to the local café requires at least minimal make-up, well-groomed hair and a 'casual' outfit that would stop traffic in other countries.

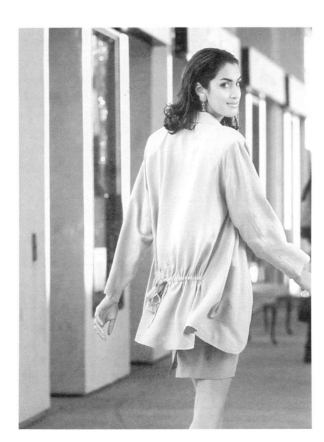

Italian women are credited with having the most natural style

Italian women love to discuss style and are forthcoming about what they think looks good and what is terrible. Where French women keep their beauty secrets to themselves, Italian women can't wait to share them with their girlfriends. When I was working in Rome I remember admiring a beautiful suit in an over-priced boutique. Another shopper had seen me slowly succumbing, almost ready to buy, when she whisked me outside to tell me where I could buy it at a discount. We hadn't exchanged more than a cursory greeting in the shop but that was enough to establish solidarity and to share a vital shopping tip.

Italian women rely on the inspiration of designers, pop groups and block buster films to see how to put things together. Anything that they consider too eccentric, irrational or outrageous is dismissed as *'molto inglese'* (very English).

Travel Tips

Despite a few notable exceptions, you won't come across many women in top management positions. So, if travelling to Italy on business you'll dress for the men, that is, their expectations if you are a businesswoman. The social pressure for women to stay home and rear families is greater than in any other European country: only 38 per cent of women work outside the home.

The relaxed social life and general openness of the people belies the formality you will meet in business. You are advised to dress as you would in London or Frankfurt but to take care that your look appeals to the Italian obsession with good design. Wear the best shoes, belt and handbag you own. Only real gold will do in Italy, so put away the fakes and buy or borrow some genuine gold earrings for the trip. Italians can spot the real thing from a distance.

The evening requires more thought and effort, even if dining with business colleagues in a restaurant. It's very easy for businesswomen to look drab and boring after six because the other women have been working for hours to create that special evening sparkle. So, just touching up your make-up won't do. You will need to change, to wear fabrics with a sheen (for example, satin or silk), and to sparkle – add the diamanté brooch or earrings.

SCANDINAVIA

It's unfair to take a broad brush to this rich, diverse region of Northern Europe. To suggest that people dress the same in darkest Lapland and in cosmopolitan Copenhagen would be ridiculous. But there are elements of style that pervade most of the region, which includes: Denmark, Sweden, Norway, Finland and Iceland.

First and foremost, Scandinavian style is contingent upon the climate. For six months of the year, when much of the region is dark and Arctic, they are bundled up sensibly from head to toe. You rarely see a woman's leg. In summer, when the sun shines incessantly for up to 24 hours a day, they wear the absolute minimum. The public gardens and parks are alive with men, women and children in minimal clothing, soaking up the sunshine.

I remember travelling to Copenhagen to launch *Color Me Beautiful* in February 1985. I wore a smart, Chanel-style suit which had served me well for similar presentations in Britain and Germany. At our Press Conference the journalists all turned up in trousers, large woollen jumpers, colourful scarves and lined boots. In my 'formal' suit, tights and high heels, I suddenly looked ridiculously inappropriate for the climate and their relaxed style. Even in business, most women wear trouser suits year round.

Feminism has a lot to answer for in Scandinavia. Perhaps in no other region are women more 'liberated', more 'equal'. But with all the fairness of the sexes is also the expectation that women should, and do, haul things around. There are no such things as porters in hotels, at the airports or train stations. Few, in Scandinavia, work in service jobs like portering!

But as a result of all their 'equal' treatment, alas, Scandinavian women have lost some of their poise. It's near impossible to walk elegantly laden down with heavy cargo. No wonder there's no market for high heels in the region. They need flat shoes to lug their shopping, carry their cases and stack their crates. There is much call upon our consultants to teach these women how to walk as well as how to dress!

At Their Best

Scandinavian women are a colourful lot. Perhaps it's due to the lack of natural sunshine for so much of the year that they love colour and wear it with such great confidence from head to toe. It cheers them up during those long, dark winters and helps them to keep going in the summer time when neither they nor the sun ever rest.

Entertaining in Scandinavia is never formal. Since they are such an egalitarian culture, the subtleties of class and snobbery are lost on them. Despite the generally high standard of living, they aren't at all pretentious and spurn conspicuous ostentation. Designer labels are lost on most Scandinavians because their restrictive import duties make most non-regional designers prohibitive in price.

For dinner, Scandinavians prefer to entertain you at home rather than in a restaurant. Women of every age and size might don an elaborate jumpsuit or some original creation with interesting details. They love to mix texture such as angora and leather; sequins and suede; wool and satin. Long, simple black hostess skirts are often teamed with a striking blouse or a hand-painted jacket with stunning results.

Travel Tips

Footwear dictates your wardrobe. In summer, keep your shoes casual – espadrilles, trainers or low wedgies. In winter, it's boots all the time. If you plan to do any walking, whether in the cobbled city centres of Copenhagen, Stockholm, Oslo, Helsinki or Reykjavik, or through mountain villages or farmlands, opt for comfort and practicality first.

Working from the feet up, choose trousers, culottes, shorts or comfortable skirts to team with your shoes. Bring one striking, colourful jacket for evenings – and layers to be added for warmth, or discarded as needed.

For business, if you don't have a smart trouser suit, consider wearing an attractive knit dress with a jacket and boots. If your working wardrobe is mainly neutral in colour, add a colourful woollen shawl to brighten it up. You can score a lot of extra points by wearing interesting jewellery – which is in short supply in Scandinavia.

THE NETHERLANDS

Perhaps the most open, tolerant and international nation in Europe is the Netherlands. Since their territory is slowly but steadily being reclaimed by the sea they have been forced into an interdependence, especially economically, with the rest of the EEC. Along with the Danes, the Dutch speak more foreign languages than any other nationality. On average they are fluent in three additional languages (English, German and French), with many modestly proficient also in several others.

The Dutch women, like the Scandinavians, are a liberated lot and stride about with purpose if not elegance; rubber soles are to be found on business as well as evening shoes. When in doubt the Dutch women wear black patent leather heels, any time of the year, which to this biased observer often kills their look.

The Dutch emulate both German design and lifestyle and buy their fashions enthusiastically in preference to French or Italian clothes. Accessories are fun and not necessarily real. Like the Belgians, the Dutch wince at the sight of women wearing diamonds during the day – New Yorkers take note.

Travel Tips

A simple, compact wardrobe of co-ordinated pieces will do you well when travelling to the Netherlands. The straighforward Dutch are suspicious of ostentation, or people who appear to care too much about their appearance. In both business and social life, dress is far less formal than in other parts of Europe, so be careful not to overdress. (In many companies the men wear sports jackets and the women wear trousers.) If travelling to the Netherlands on business, opt for the smart but understated rather than something at the cutting edge of fashion. Excessive effort to co-ordinate accessories will work against you here.

For evening, matt fabrics are recommended over shiny or elaborate texture, since Dutch entertainment is warm and familiar rather than stiff and formal.

Despite the openness of society and the early liberation of women, Dutch businessmen are among the most chauvinistic you'll ever meet. As in Italy, there's terrific pressure for women to give up their careers and be wives and mothers full-time until the children are fully grown. Only recently are younger women trying to keep their work and have children at the same time. With few women in senior positions, Dutch men find it difficult to accept other women from abroad who have power. So wield yours with finesse and charm rather than lock horns; otherwise you'll run out of puff when up against their stubborn resistance.

GREAT BRITAIN

You might have to fret over your nails in New York, worry about your proportions being current in Paris and your labels getting recognised in Rome, but when it comes to travelling to Britain all the pressure is off. Nowhere else in Europe has such eclecticism as well as understatement in style as the UK. Those who have money may dress as if they have none and those without may spend their last pound on a new lipstick.

Brace yourself for a spectrum of style. In London fewer women 'dress-up' as if they were in a capital city like Paris, New York or Rome but dash about as if they've just popped out for a pint of milk. Those who are well-dressed in Britain are mainly foreign with the natives feeling they have much more sensible things to spend their money on than clothes.

Non-working women have a spending priority list a mile long. At the bottom a postscript might appear noting a 'frock needed for drinks party'. They will splash out for top of the line interior fabrics and 'soft-furnishings' but may well balk over paying £30.00 for a pair of shoes. Here's a sweeping generalisation (and an explanation) for you: whereas the Frenchman is prepared to devote a percentage of his income for his wife's wardrobe – after all, she's a vital asset to his success – British men tend to be less clothes conscious. So, many housewives don't have a dress allowance. Their 'housekeeping' money also has to cover clothing.

Working women do now spend money on clothes, as being well-dressed in business becomes increasingly important as well as competitive. But guilt complexes handed down from their mothers still preclude many working women from spending on quality. Many play it safe, buying from the national institution, 'Marks & Spencer', and never make it beyond there.

Despite a deservedly high reputation for producing gifted young designers and innovative styles, as a fashion capital London trails behind Paris, Milan, New York and Tokyo. At the extreme ends of the fashion spectrum from basic country clothes to wild party frocks, Britain is a leader, but everyday clothes can be rather patchy. If looking for a smart, yet different suit for work, you'll probably find yourself putting German, French, Italian or even Irish (Paul Costello to be exact) before traditional British manufacturers.

Travel Tips

The ultimate sin in Britain, whether for business or social events, is to be overdressed. If in doubt about the style of an occasion, play it safe. For a dinner party, a simple yet elegant short dress with classic accessories is recommended.

Save your exciting bright colours for when you are surer of your standing and the event. Use basic colours in quality fabrics instead. Do wear make-up but, again, if you don't know your hosts stick to neutral tones.

In business it's not difficult to make an impact simply by looking your best and well-groomed. You will find that despite a long-standing reputation for reserve, the British deserve a lot more credit for their charm, wit and good humour. You'll never enjoy doing business as much as you can in Britain. To score points with the British be self-deprecating and don't discuss money – as in: 'Oh you like my necklace. Well, it cost a fortune!' Such openness is considered rather vulgar by these very civilised folk.

UNITED STATES

Visitors to America are struck by the diversity of looks as they compare regions of this vast continent. Climate has something to do with the fact that Californians dress differently from folks in the Mid-West or Northeast. But also, each geographic region has its own culture and lifestyle that are as diverse from one another as the Scottish are from the Italians or the Spanish from the Germans.

However, you do see a great similarity of dress around America. A shopping mall anywhere in the States will be thronged with women in brightly coloured track suits. At rush hour in major city streets, smartly suited women stride exuberantly to and from their offices, sporting trainers, walkmans and 'backpack' attaches. Formal evening parties welcome women in short or long dresses, trousers or skirts.

It's too simple to broad brush America by saying 'anything goes'. Each region has a flair and subtle style code of its own. Here are a few insights for you to consider before venturing to America on business or pleasure.

The Northeast Corridor (from New England, New York, New Jersey and Pennsylvania to Washington D.C.)

To Europeans, the Northeast is the most classic, conservative understated style region in all of America. It is here that the preppy look was born and survives generation after generation with women wearing minimal make-up, A-line skirts and sensible, unstylish shoes. British travellers feel very much at home here with average women (excluding the New York and New Jersey area) preferring understatement to glitz.

New York, America's fashion capital, sets the tone. Its inhabitants invest heavily every season in the latest looks; whether they pay the full price or do well at one of the many 'designer outlets' in the Northeast, these women want to look *now*. By 'designer', Americans simply mean expensive off-the-peg – not couture. Looks are bought in toto from one designer as it is important for others to be able to tally up the value of the clothes on their backs. If Donna Karan, Calvin Klein or Ralph Lauren says this is how the outfit is to be worn, this is how they wear it.

Nail salons are more common than hair salons, particularly in New York. When visiting you must give it a go, if only for the entertainment. As you ponder how you'll ever be able to wash dishes again, with long red lacquered claws cemented to your fingers, you'll overhear everyone's social adventures from the night before in glittering detail.

If on business, be prepared to be outdone by New Yorkers who have a wide range of exciting choices in business clothes at very reasonable prices. Stroll down Fifth Avenue and just look at the women. The perennial success of Klein, Karan and Lauren who produce simple styles in luscious neutrals mean it's probably best to play down bright colours for quality, understated classics.

The Mid-West

Chicago is the business capital of Middle America, and more friendly, open and bearable than New York. Even though a huge city, it is suburban in style. Most people who commute from well-manicured surrounding towns aren't into big city glamour. The harsh winters dictate sensible style: lined boots, down-feather coats, and woollen hats.

There's no need to compete with Mid-Westerners in style, the people are simply too nice and egalitarian. Save the effort for New York. Here, be yourself; they'll like you for it.

The South

There's the old south and the new south. The old southerner was born and bred in the region and is more genteel than the 'upstarts' who have moved here from the other parts for a better climate, more relaxed lifestyle and higher standard of living.

If visiting 'old southerners' be prepared for a formality that is almost European. Unlike other parts of the States, they'll use seating plans at dinner and be charmed if you circulate and spread your foreign charm amongst the guests.

New southerners, who are found en masse in Atlanta, Miami or Orlando, have a penchant for blinding colour. The bright sunshine of the region allows them to use more colour than in more northern states, but they do get carried away. If visiting on business, wear the brightest blouse you own with your suit. Neutrals would be too severe.

The warm, humid southern climate means that blended fabrics – part-natural, part-manmade – are most practical. Choose washable tops and blouses as they will need freshening after every wearing. Softer, light hosiery is required in a light denier.

The South-West (specifically Texas)

Texans refuse to admit it but the 1980s TV series *Dallas* did convey how important style is to these charming, larger than life Americans. The pressure on working women is terrific, but they find time to spend 'heaps' of money on looking good.

Texan and French women share a love of beautiful hair, but their styles are diametrically apart. French chic is all about a well cut, manageable style, whilst Texan hair is all about lots of volume.

If travelling to the South-West, make an effort with your hair – if it is short, fluff it out with some spray. Be more adventurous with your eyeshadows and lipsticks, too; never garish, simply more colourful.

Dining out is either diamanté and silk, or denim and cowboy boots. Bring a good casual outfit – an interesting blouse to team with a skirt or trousers. Then soften your classics with interesting accessories, to be feminine without losing your professionalism.

The West (specifically California)

In California, individuality is more important than in New York. Perhaps less concerned about what's in style, Californians enjoy looking good and being relaxed.

Women in business are smartly suited but use accessories that make visitors do a double-take. (Brooches the size of TV sets were very popular last year.) Californians don't like packaged looks and need to express themselves no matter be they a beach bum or a banker.

Serious high heels are laughable to Californians, so wear mid-high styles for best effect. Look out for beautiful, but very reasonably priced, silk T-shirts in subtle 'sherbert' shades as well as luminous brights.

Enjoying such a wonderful climate, living is very 'outdoor' in California and hence more relaxed. If invited to dinner, dress-down. Wear trousers, soft culottes or a flowing skirt in your best colours with fun accessories.

Travel is mainly by car so take knits and jerseys that can endure the journeys rather than natural fibres that can crease excessively.

AUSTRALIA AND NEW ZEALAND

The wonderful climate in the Pacific Basin means that most Australians and New Zealanders enjoy an active, outdoor life, and dress accordingly. Skirts are loose and long or abandoned for shorts. Europeans lucky enough to travel down under during their winter and the Australians' summer find the contrast in lifestyle so startling that they're not quite sure if the jet lag is worse than the cultural shock.

With economies linked to the land, sheep farming in particular, natural fibres reign supreme. Manmade stuff is available but at horrific prices since import tariffs are so high on foreign textiles. But the Aussies hanker after creaseproof fabrics and often don't appreciate how lucky they are to be surrounded by such wonderful natural fibre fashions.

Styles are more akin to southern California, due to lifestyle, climate and pervasive American influences in films and imports, than any harking back to a

European past. As a member of the Commonwealth, British fashion is more important than comparable offerings from Italy, France or Germany – no doubt due to favourable tariffs on imports.

Travel Tips

The high humidity prevalent for many months of the year makes it pointless to wear a lot of make-up as it will become a sweaty mess after an hour. Opt instead for a sunblock tinted moisturiser, natural-looking eye make-up and lipstick.

In business, the women are surprisingly smart. I say surprisingly because the contrast with their casual style is pronounced. They really 'dress-up' for work and have a penchant for shiny blouses with business suits. Their hair looks terrific and they always accessorise with vigour never caution.

To score points with Australians try and relax. Their natural passion for wanderlust means they'll be eager to share stories of when they visited your country or will be keen for tips on where to stay and what to see for a forthcoming adventure. As with many Americans, the subtleties of European status are lost on Australians. They'll take you for who you are rather than who your parents might be, or the kudos understood in Europe about having gone to the right schools or being a member of some exclusive club. Here you can let your hair down and will no doubt return a different person for the experience.

Confident body talk

SO far we've discussed your image in terms of your appearance and how to develop your personal style. But no matter how well-dressed you are, whether at work or out socially, if you don't convey natural confidence through your body language then your image will suffer.

Let's go back to those statistics about the impact of your image. Remember, 55% of the impression you make on others depends on how you look *and* how you act.

Even before you open your mouth to introduce yourself, people have already made judgements about you. From how you look in terms of your personal style – choice of clothing and colours – they'll decide how successful you are, where you might live, how old you are. By how you act they'll form a first impression about your confidence, your honesty, your personality. How you walk, enter a room, shake hands, use eye contact, facial expression and gestures convey more than you realise about your personality.

If in doubt, we believe others' body language rather than their words. Think of a politician when handling difficult questions from an aggressive journalist on television. Why is it you can always tell when a public official is being economical with the truth? We notice that under stress his eyes begin darting hurriedly from side to side. He instinctively starts rubbing his nose and upper lip area, almost as if to cover his mouth, to prevent the untruths from escaping. If standing he might shift from one foot to the other or instinctively cross his arms as if to protect himself from the barrage of unwelcome inquiry.

Remember the last dinner party you attended, when you met someone and really rubbed each other up the wrong way. You simply couldn't find common ground for discussion and bored each other to tears. Think of when you said good night upon leaving. No doubt you smiled, shook hands and said 'lovely to meet you'. You both knew that the pleasant and polite salutation was a lie. Was it the false smile? You know the ones when the lips move but the rest of the face, particularly the eyes, remains frozen. The face actually says, 'it darn well wasn't so lovely to meet you!'

A job interview doesn't begin when you are seated comfortably across the desk of the personnel manager, but when you first walk into his or her office. From that moment on the interviewer's brain is registering signals about you – your confidence, your energy, your abilities. Think of the last time you were interviewed or met someone new. What non-verbal signals do you think you sent out? And what non-verbal signs did you pick up from the other person? What I'd like to cover in the next few pages are the key things you should be aware of about your behaviour signals at work and in new, stressful situations. The focus will be on using your behaviour to express yourself and your personality, and to appear confident. Many of the situations come from experience shared by my clients who've been caught in unknown territory, particularly with men in business, and didn't know what to do. I want to prepare you for the unknown for you to send only right, positive signals.

HANDSHAKES

One of the strongest personal signals you send about yourself every day is through your handshake. How you shake hands tells others three things about you:

- how confident you are
- how sheltered a life you lead
- how much respect you have for others.

You express confidence through your handshake in two ways. First, by how quickly you offer your hand upon meeting people. Hesitation conveys uncertainty and lack of confidence. And second, by the firmness of your grip: if it's weak you are unsure of yourself; if it's too firm you're overconfident and egotistical; if it's firm and direct then you are telling others that you know who you are.

Handshakes also tell others if you've travelled a lot or live a rather sheltered life where you socialise with only very familiar friends. Through working or travelling abroad and in situations where you are meeting new people all the time, you grow accustomed to shaking hands and can do so without any stress. Women who rarely shake hands can find doing so very scary and need some tutoring and practice to develop a confident handshake.

Your handshake also expresses the amount of respect you hold for others. If, when approaching a group, you only shake the hands of a few and ignore the rest you are sending clear signals that the remaining cast aren't as important in your estimation.

Making the Right Impression

Think of the last time you shook someone's hand that really left a bad impression. You know the ones: the limp, wet fish; the power-hungry, bone-crusher; the patronising finger-tip tweeter. Needless to say you don't want a handshake like any of these.

Aim for a firm, direct grip so that the 'web' between your thumb and forefinger meets that of your partner. Anything halfway is a sign of weakness. Anything more is too threatening.

If you have sweaty palms, don't despair. Many women as well as men have moist palms, particularly when nervous. If prone to sweaty palms, spray them (palms only) with an anti-perspirant before a meeting.

Always offer your hand when meeting someone new. In Europe, if you don't offer your hand to a man he won't extend his to you out of traditional politeness. In business, if you fail to extend a hand to other executives, whether male or female, you'll lose credibility.

PERSONAL TERRITORY

Everyone has a personal territory or comfort zone, an area of space around ourselves which we like to keep clear. With friends, family and loved ones we don't require the same amount of space as we do with people we meet for the first time. But we require more space or distance from people we feel threatened by. Edward Hall, an American anthropologist, was a pioneer in defining what man's spacial needs are. His 1960s research into the proximity we feel comfortable with in different cultures and situations has helped many understand their own comfort zone and, more importantly, interpret others'.

As an American from a large family I have a very small personal territory. I like to be near people, to touch. When I first moved to Britain, I overwhelmed many people by getting too close. I remember talking to a group of women at a cocktail party and I touched one woman on the upper arm to convey understanding. Her whole body stiffened, she stepped back and cut off eye contact. I had invaded her personal zone and had made her feel uncomfortable. Ever since then I have resisted my own inclination to get near people and to respect the space they require from which to communicate.

How Big Is Your Bubble?

Your personal bubble or comfort zone is determined by where you grew up and the density of population. Across cultures, even within countries there are wide distinctions in personal bubbles. Upon meeting a Swede for the first time you appreciate that most keep a wide distance, up to 4 feet (1.22m) after having met and shaken hands, even when just making small talk. In contrast, most Italians are terribly offended if you don't stay close by. To retreat by up to 4 feet after meeting is a great insult.

But within cultures there are also variations. In Paris, even though it's a large, bustling city with lots of people, the natives have big bubbles. Travel south to Cannes and someone born and bred on the Côte d'Azur needs very little space and draws you physically near.

Allan Pease, an Australian Management Consultant who lectures on cross-cultural body language, defines the comfort zones at work in most Western societies as:

- The Intimate Zone is between 6–18 inches (15–45cm). Into this 'bubble' we allow only our nearest and dearest.

- The Personal Zone is between 18 inches–4 feet (45cm–1.22m). This is the bubble we create at work, and on social occasions.

- The Social Zone is between 4–12 feet (1.22–3.6m) and is a larger bubble we require when interacting with people we don't know very well; for example, the woman collecting for charity, the shopkeeper.

- The Public Zone is over 12 feet (3.6m). This much larger bubble is needed when we address a group of unknown people.

A good way to find out the size of your bubble is to watch how comfortable you feel the next time you are at a cocktail party. Do you step back and create more space for yourself, and feel hemmed in if people get too close? Or don't you mind it if people crowd near.

Also, try experimenting with other people's bubbles. Occasionally, I like playing a cat and mouse at my seminars. I'll ask for someone who grew up in Scandinavia (where they have very large bubbles) and for someone who was raised in Italy or Spain (who have smaller bubbles). I'll stand the two volunteers far apart at the front of the room and slowly walk towards them. When I approach the Scandinavian he steps back as soon as I approach about 4 feet (1.22m) away from him. By contrast, the Italian or Spanish bred volunteer lets me come as close as 2 feet before they start to shuffle and fidget indicating: far enough.

The point of knowing the area of your own personal territory and learning to recognise other people's is that it's important to make others feel comfortable around you. If you have a large bubble and others you meet have smaller ones, take a deep breath and appreciate that they aren't trying to 'attack' you, they just need to get closer to communicate. If you are selling yourself or your company it's important for you to put up with a little discomfort to make a client feel more at ease. Only return to your own bubble – by stepping back – if a man consciously or unconsciously takes advantage of your space in or outside the business environment.

ON THE DEFENSIVE: UNWELCOME MANOEUVRES

There are situations when people, especially men, test your nerve by using aggressive or sexual advances. Unwelcome manoeuvres come in many forms, ranging from the very subtle, like the invasion of your territory, to perplexing and awkward, like the kiss rather than the preferred handshake greeting.

It's a wise woman who has thought through how she'd deal with awkward situations before they actually happen. So even if these examples of unwelcome manoeuvres haven't happened to you as yet, think through how you would handle a comparable situation. I'll use examples that women have shared with me and which seem to occur, at every level of business, with such frequency that they merit every woman's attention.

When Your Turf's Invaded

Male and female colleagues can undermine you at work by intentionally or unwittingly invading your space. When someone sits on your desk as you are seated, looks over your shoulder as you are working, or simply moves in too closely when you're seated or standing, you feel vulnerable and threatened. Hold your ground by using the following tactics:

- If someone gets too close by leaning against your side, a method used to either dominate or threaten, swiftly turn and face them, then step back. If you have a file or some papers in hand hold them up between you as a barrier. Cut the conversation short and leave.

- When someone sits on your desk or comes in from behind to look over your shoulder, stand-up, face them then walk slowly towards them. This usually causes the predator to retreat backwards, reversing the power threat from him or her to you.

The Unwelcome Kiss

In European countries, like France, Italy and Spain, businesswomen need to be prepared for a kiss greeting on the second or third meeting. But rarely is this more than a tasteful cheek-to-cheek number without body contact. British and American women find this difficult to get used to and worry about losing power when they accept a kiss. My advice is accept it gracefully and explain to any male colleagues travelling with you that you've made a cultural concession, 'when in Rome . . .' to forestall any boorish rumours starting back at the office.

If you wish to greet a male colleague with something more familiar than a handshake but less so than a kiss, try a warm, but businesslike touch to his upper arm. This works quite well if your salutation is also less formal; for example: 'You're looking well, Paul,' or, when leaving: 'See you soon, Helmut.'

Forestalling the Smacker

When you see the Slobbering Smacker approaching a different strategy is required. Switch on the 'arm lever' – a sharp forward propulsion of the right arm that extends a firm handshake but keeps the arm rigid, clearly signalling 'Keep Your Distance'. If your left hand is unencumbered, bring it up to his right shoulder as you shake hands for a full barrier, and with a gentle push direct him to where you want him to go – literally speaking, that is.

MAKING AN ENTRANCE

How you walk through the door tells us whether or not you believe in yourself and whether or not others should believe in you.

So don't hesitate, hold your head up, take a deep breath and go in with purpose in your pace and a smile on your face. Don't encumber yourself with anything more than a briefcase (in business) or a handbag. Make sure if you wear a coat that it does your all-important entrance justice. If yours isn't up to par, take it off and carry it, folded, over your left arm (the same one carrying your briefcase), leaving your right hand free to make handshakes.

EYE CONTACT: PRACTICE HELPS

Perhaps the most obvious sign of self-consciousness is the inability to look people in the eye for prolonged periods when communicating. Eye contact reveals a lot about you – your honesty or hostility, your enthusiasm or disinterest. If you can't look people in the eye, you appear to be underconfident, concealing something, or just not attending to what is being said.

The answer is *not* to develop an unrelenting gaze because that sort of eye contact conveys arrogance or hostility. The aim is to strike a balance between the two extremes – alternating brief periods of eye-to-eye contact and briefly shifting your gaze.

Anyone can improve their eye contact through practice. The best place to start is with friends, family and especially children. Watch how you can improve a child's attention if you read him a story with intermittent eye contact versus no eye contact. When shopping, try engaging the sales assistants with strong eye contact – you'll see their service and manner improve!

When speaking to more than one person at a time, remember to 'connect' with everyone in turn via eye contact. I love speaking to large groups and working my way through different parts of the audience with direct eye contact. It's amazing how much more attentive an audience you will have when you connect in this way, non-verbally, with the eyes.

TELLING GESTURES

You know instinctively when you're not getting through to people, when they are bored or negative. Even if they say positive things like 'that sounds interesting', or 'what a good idea', their gestures belie their words. If someone says something favourable and their arms are crossed, they are probably thinking the reverse; unless, of course, a gust of cold air just caught them and they're warming themselves against the chill.

When you are feeling nervous or negative and find yourself adopting a crossed arm pose (or closed body gesture as it is known by body language experts), try holding something, a file or some papers in the bend of one arm. This will act as a partial 'shield', to make you feel more comfortable and to come across as less hostile or defensive.

'Holding Your Own Hands' in front or behind your body is another negative, closed gesture implying weakness or nervousness when addressing people. Try holding a pen in one hand or putting one hand in a side pocket, if you are are too nervous to adopt the preferred stance of both hands at the side – the most open and confident posture. Once you've got over the first few sentences, and begin using gestures to emphasis your points you'll feel more relaxed.

A *fit image*

HEALTH and fitness are vital to your image, because a fit woman sparkles. Her vitality comes through her eyes, the glow of her skin, the lilt in her walk. So don't allow yourself to become sluggish and drawn from a poor diet, lack of exercise or insufficient rest. These are all preventable. Being over 30 and having had children or a demanding career are not good reasons for opting out on fitness. You want to be strong and healthy not only to look good but, more importantly, to cope well with the demands of modern living.

Ponder a minute the state of your fitness:

- Do you know how much food your body requires each day to function efficiently?

- Can you remember what you had for dinner last night?

- Could you climb a flight of stairs briskly without puffing when you hit the top?

- Do you feel and look bloated other than during your period?

- If you work, do you feel sluggish after lunch?

- Has your figure changed dramatically for the worse in the last 10 years?

- Do you know how to lose weight and inches when you want to?

- Are you flexible and limber? Can you sit on the floor and stretch out easily and without strain?

- Do you wish you had more stamina?

- Can you release tension and sleep soundly to awake refreshed each morning?

THINK TRIM NOT SLIM

Correct weight is only a part of being fit. You and your doctor are the best judges of what might be best for you depending upon your height, bone structure and age. Unfortunately standard charts produced by the medical profession don't account for bone structure. If you are small boned, deduct 6lb (2.7kg); if you are large boned, add an extra 6lb (2.7kg) (see page 86). But don't be overly concerned about weight unless it affects your health and you need to set targets to lose pounds on your doctor's orders. If you are around normal weight, aim for trimming up rather than slimming down. By trimming up with exercise you can lose inches where you most want to in order to wear clothes more comfortably and attractively.

Before undertaking any exercise routine, if it's been a while since you engaged in any such activity do consult your doctor first to see if there are any reasons why you need to take care. However, gentle activities like walking and swimming are two of the best aerobic exercises and require no medical approval – only a will to get moving.

If you've already been exercising for some time – especially with weights or high-impact aerobics – it would be wise to consult an osteopath to see if you are still properly aligned or if you are overstressing any joints or ligaments.

I know it's difficult to start exercising and reform bad habits, but you simply have no choice unless you want to look and feel older than you need and not be able to enjoy life to the fullest. Don't panic. I'm not going to suggest marathon training for the uninitiated. But we all need to work on both our aerobic endurance and our flexibility in order to look and feel our best.

The pluses of exercise are many. You enhance your stamina, your flexibility and your energy. After a good brisk walk all the tensions of the day disappear. You'll wonder what you were worried about beforehand. You develop strength. All women need to be strong – as strong physically as we are mentally and emotionally. A good workout – whether it be a bike ride, ice skating, a swim or more organised pursuits like squash, tennis, aerobics or skiing – also banishes the blues. Yes, working up a good sweat brings you right out of yourself and gives you a 'high' which is equivalent to or better than good sex.

CHOOSE A PROGRAMME TO SUIT YOU

Some women who are very disciplined find exercising at home, alone, with the help of a videotape best. They enjoy the privacy and the ability to build up their strength at their own pace. The only problem is that we usually don't push ourselves as hard or develop as well on our own as we do with the encouragement of an instructor and working alongside other women with similar goals.

Joining an exercise club can be daunting. Everyone seems to look younger and slimmer than you are. And when you first sign-on you can feel a real outsider if there are cliques. If that is your first experience – don't give up. There are good exercise groups or clubs which make an effort to welcome newcomers and ensure that you develop at your own pace.

The more regularly you attend, at least twice a week, the sooner you'll feel part of the group and once you make friends, you will realise that all the other women have the same insecurities about their bodies that you do.

A successful exercise programme needs to suit you, to be one you can really enjoy and carry out regularly. A week shouldn't go by without you being able to list five active things you've done for a minimum of 20 minutes at a time. Walking more is the best way to start, while you consider more organised ways to get fit. Get off the train two stops before you need to and walk the extra distance to the office – briskly but not so quickly that you get out of breath. Take the stairs rather than escalators or lifts in department stores. Try swimming once a week. Do bum squeezes as you sit at your desk, when driving or when standing waiting for the bus. Avoid exercise routines or sporting activities that require elaborate preparation or expensive gear – at least until you know you are really committed. To start with it's a matter of trial and error; some women love jazz classes while others prefer stretch ones. Discover what's right for you and make a commitment to do it on a regular basis.

Cherish your body, protect it, nurture it by eating properly, by exercising and by taking time to relax so that you always have a confident, fit image.

IN CONCLUSION

Together, we've charted a course through that fascinating subject of 'Your Image'. You've learned why it's important to value yourself and to project yourself well to others in your personal and professional lives. There are plenty of guidelines and valuable advice for you to reflect on and select from as you develop your own personal style.

If you haven't already done so, prepare a plan for investing in yourself. How much can you afford (or not afford!) to spend? What should be your priorities? Is it a new hairstyle or a fresh approach to doing your make-up that would make the greatest impact? Or are the colours in your current wardrobe simply too safe and predictable? Perhaps the best medicine for your new image would be a couple of new blouses in your favourite seasonal colours to boost your morale and win compliments from others.

Remember to walk before you run. Take your personal image development one step at a time. Explore and experiment before you make any final choices. Treat yourself to an afternoon, when the stores aren't crowded with harried shoppers, and just try on some new colours and styles. Leave your cheque book at home if you think you might get carried away!

Do an audit of your existing wardrobe and get rid of all the clutter that's letting your image down. Focus on three new things you really need this season to envigorate the rest of your wardrobe. Is it a jacket, a pair of shoes or earrings, a new scarf in your colours, or a more current skirt or pair of trousers?

As your Image Consultant, all I can do now is leave you with this rich source of ideas, and let *you* decide on how to make more – the most – of yourself. If in developing your new image you feel more confident both in being and expressing yourself, then I will consider my efforts to have been worthwhile. I hope you do too!

The seasonal palettes in full

ON the following pages are complete lists of the best colours for each Seasonal Type. These colours are a guideline to help you when shopping. Be sure any new purchase co-ordinates with at least three other items in your wardrobe. See page 191 for details about purchasing fabric swatches in your seasonal colours; swatches can be an invaluable reminder of your colours when shopping.

Clear Spring Palette	Warm Spring Palette	Light Spring Palette
1 Navy	1 Camel	1 Camel
2 Light Grey	2 Khaki	2 Khaki
3 Medium Grey	3 Bronze	3 Pewter
4 Charcoal	4 Golden brown	4 Light grey
5 Black	5 Dark brown	5 Medium grey
6 Black brown	6 Gold	6 Blue charcoal
7 Soft white	7 Ivory	7 Soft white
8 Ivory	8 Cream	8 Ivory
9 Stone	9 Stone	9 Stone
10 Taupe	10 Taupe	10 Taupe
11 Pewter	11 Grey green	11 Light peach
12 Silver	12 Medium grey	12 Warm pastel pink
13 Icy blue	13 Light peach	13 Powder pink
14 Icy violet	14 Peach	14 Peach
15 Warm pastel pink	15 Deep peach	15 Clear salmon
16 Clear salmon	16 Light orange	16 Coral
17 Coral	17 Clear salmon	17 Light orange
18 Coral pink	18 Coral	18 Mango
19 Warm pink	19 Mango	19 Rose pink
20 Mango	20 Tomato red	20 Coral pink
21 Deep rose	21 Terracotta	21 Warm pink
22 Hot pink	22 Marigold	22 Deep rose
23 Clear red	23 Pumpkin	23 Watermelon
24 True red	24 Rust	24 Clear red
25 Light clear gold	25 Buttermilk	25 Buttermilk
26 Lemon yellow	26 Buff	26 Buff
27 Bright golden yellow	27 Light clear gold	27 Light clear gold

Clear Spring Palette

28 Mint
29 Pastel yellow green
30 Gold
31 Emerald turquoise
32 Kelly green
33 True green
34 Emerald green
35 Forest green
36 Olive
37 Light teal
38 Clear teal
39 Chinese blue
40 Clear aqua
41 Hot turquoise
42 Violet
43 Purple
44 Periwinkle
45 Deep periwinkle
46 Bright periwinkle
47 Medium blue
48 True blue

Warm Spring Palette

28 Bright golden yellow
29 Yellow gold
30 Bright yellow green
31 Mint
32 Pastel yellow green
33 Light true green
34 Lime
35 Light moss
36 Moss
37 Light aqua
38 Clear aqua
39 Light teal
40 Turquoise
41 Emerald turquoise
42 Jade
43 Medium blue
44 Deep periwinkle
45 Violet
46 Purple
47 Light navy
48 Teal

Light Spring Palette

28 Bright golden yellow
29 Pastel yellow green
30 Light moss
31 Bright yellow green
32 Blue green
33 Emerald turquoise
34 Light teal
35 Clear aqua
36 Light aqua
37 Mint
38 Powder blue
39 Light lavender
40 Sky blue
41 Periwinkle
42 Purple
43 Violet
44 Light navy
45 True blue
46 Medium blue
47 Silver
48 Gold

Light Summer Palette

1 Light grey
2 Grey blue
3 Medium grey
4 Pewter
5 Cocoa
6 Rose brown
7 Soft white
8 Ivory
9 Rose beige
10 Stone
11 Taupe
12 Gold
13 Warm pastel pink
14 Powder pink
15 Clear salmon
16 Rose pink
17 Rose
18 Silver
19 Coral pink
20 Warm pink
21 Mango
22 Deep rose
23 Watermelon
24 Clear red
25 Buttermilk
26 Light lemon yellow
27 Mint
28 Pastel blue green
29 Light aqua
30 Clear aqua
31 Blue green
32 Emerald turquoise
33 Light teal
34 Soft teal
35 Spruce

Cool Summer Palette

1 Light grey
2 Medium grey
3 Blue charcoal
4 Grey blue
5 Charcoal
6 Pewter
7 Soft white
8 Rose beige
9 Stone
10 Taupe
11 Cocoa
12 Rose brown
13 Icy pink
14 Dusty rose
15 Rose pink
16 Orchid
17 Hot pink
18 Soft fuchsia
19 Deep rose
20 True red
21 Blue red
22 Watermelon
23 Raspberry
24 Burgundy
25 Light true green
26 Emerald turquoise
27 Teal
28 Soft teal
29 Spruce
30 Pine
31 Light lemon yellow
32 Mint
33 Medium aqua
34 Clear aqua
35 Hot turquoise

Soft Summer Palette

1 Light grey
2 Medium grey
3 Grey green
4 Pewter
5 Coffee brown
6 Rose brown
7 Soft white
8 Ivory
9 Rose beige
10 Stone
11 Taupe
12 Cocoa
13 Powder pink
14 Dusty rose
15 Orchid
16 Rose pink
17 Rose
18 Soft fuchsia
19 Raspberry
20 Warm pink
21 Deep rose
22 Watermelon
23 Blue red
24 Burgundy
25 Buttermilk
26 Light lemon yellow
27 Mint
28 Pastel blue green
29 Blue green
30 Emerald turquoise
31 Turquoise
32 Jade
33 Spruce
34 Forest green
35 Soft teal

Light Summer Palette

36 Light navy
37 Lavender
38 Powder blue
39 Sky blue
40 Medium blue
41 True blue
42 Cadet blue
43 Lavender
44 Amethyst
45 Periwinkle
46 Deep periwinkle
47 Violet
48 Purple

Cool Summer Palette

36 Chinese blue
37 Sky blue
38 Lavender
39 Amethyst
40 Violet
41 Plum
42 Purple
43 Periwinkle
44 Cadet blue
45 True blue
46 Royal blue
47 Navy
48 Silver

Soft Summer Palette

36 Teal
37 Light navy
38 Grey blue
39 Charcoal
40 Cadet blue
41 Sky blue
42 Periwinkle
43 Deep periwinkle
44 Amethyst
45 Purple
46 Medium blue
47 Silver
48 Gold

Soft Autumn Palette

1 Mahogany
2 Dark brown
3 Rose brown
4 Coffee brown
5 Grey green
6 Charcoal
7 Taupe
8 Cream
9 Camel
10 Khaki
11 Pewter
12 Medium grey
13 Light peach
14 Warm pink
15 Deep rose
16 Salmon
17 Silver
18 Gold
19 Salmon pink
20 Bittersweet
21 Tomato red
22 Watermelon
23 Rust
24 Terracotta
25 Soft white
26 Ivory
27 Stone
28 Buttermilk
29 Buff
30 Light lemon yellow
31 Yellow gold
32 Mint
33 Emerald turquoise
34 Turquoise
35 Jade
36 Teal
37 Bronze
38 Moss
39 Light moss
40 Lime
41 Olive
42 Forest green
43 Cadet blue

Warm Autumn Palette

1 Camel
2 Khaki
3 Grey green
4 Golden brown
5 Coffee brown
6 Dark brown
7 Ivory
8 Cream
9 Stone
10 Taupe
11 Pewter
12 Medium grey
13 Light peach
14 Deep peach
15 Salmon
16 Salmon pink
17 Coral
18 Pumpkin
19 Terracotta
20 Tomato red
21 Bittersweet
22 Rust
23 Mahogany
24 Aubergine
25 Buttermilk
26 Buff
27 Light clear gold
28 Yellow gold
29 Light moss
30 Lime
31 Moss
32 Olive
33 Bronze
34 Mustard
35 Marigold
36 Gold
37 Turquoise
38 Emerald turquoise
39 Jade
40 Teal
41 Forest green
42 Light true green
43 Clear aqua

Deep Autumn Palette

1 Taupe
2 Pewter
3 Grey green
4 Black brown
5 Charcoal
6 Black
7 Soft white
8 Ivory
9 Cream
10 Stone
11 Camel
12 Buttermilk
13 Light peach
14 Deep peach
15 Salmon pink
16 Mango
17 Bittersweet
18 Tomato red
19 True red
20 Terracotta
21 Rust
22 Mahogany
23 Brown burgundy
24 Aubergine
25 Yellow gold
26 Marigold
27 Mustard
28 Light moss
29 Moss
30 Gold
31 Lime
32 Olive
33 Bronze
34 True green
35 Emerald green
36 Forest green
37 Mint
38 Hot turquoise
39 Chinese blue
40 Turquoise
41 Emerald turquoise
42 Pine
43 True blue

Soft Autumn Palette

44 Light navy
45 Deep periwinkle
46 Amethyst
47 Purple
48 Aubergine

Warm Autumn Palette

44 Light aqua
45 Violet
46 Deep periwinkle
47 Purple
48 Light navy

Deep Autumn Palette

44 Teal
45 Navy
46 Purple
47 Deep periwinkle
48 Silver

Deep Winter Palette

1 Black
2 Charcoal
3 Pewter
4 Black brown
5 Mahogany
6 Brown burgundy
7 Pure white
8 Soft white
9 Stone
10 Taupe
11 Icy grey
12 Medium grey
13 Hot pink
14 Raspberry
15 Magenta
16 Fuchsia
17 Cranberry
18 True red
19 Mango
20 Tomato red
21 Rust
22 Blue red
23 Burgundy
24 Aubergine
25 Mint
26 Icy green
27 Icy yellow
28 Lemon yellow
29 Icy violet
30 Icy pink
31 Turquoise
32 Emerald green
33 Forest green
34 Pine
35 Olive
36 Gold
37 True green
38 Emerald turquoise
39 Teal
40 Clear teal
41 True blue
42 Silver
43 Hot turquoise
44 Chinese blue
45 Bright periwinkle
46 Purple
47 Royal blue
48 Navy

Cool Winter Palette

1 Icy grey
2 Light grey
3 Medium grey
4 Charcoal
5 Black
6 Black brown
7 Pure white
8 Soft white
9 Stone
10 Taupe
11 Pewter
12 Silver
13 Dusty rose
14 Rose pink
15 Shocking pink
16 Hot pink
17 Fuchsia
18 Magenta
19 Deep rose
20 True red
21 Blue red
22 Raspberry
23 Cranberry
24 Burgundy
25 Mint
26 Icy green
27 Icy yellow
28 Icy blue
29 Icy violet
30 Icy pink
31 Lemon yellow
32 Blue green
33 Emerald turquoise
34 True green
35 Emerald green
36 Pine
37 Hot turquoise
38 Chinese blue
39 Clear teal
40 Teal
41 Medium blue
42 Deep periwinkle
43 Bright periwinkle
44 True blue
45 Royal blue
46 Navy
47 Purple
48 Plum

Clear Winter Palette

1 Light grey
2 Medium grey
3 Charcoal
4 Black
5 Black brown
6 Pewter
7 Pure white
8 Soft white
9 Icy yellow
10 Icy grey
11 Stone
12 Taupe
13 Icy blue
14 Icy violet
15 Icy pink
16 Shocking pink
17 Hot pink
18 Deep rose
19 Mango
20 Clear red
21 Blue red
22 True red
23 Raspberry
24 Silver
25 Fuchsia
26 Magenta
27 Cranberry
28 Burgundy
29 Aubergine
30 Gold
31 Mint
32 Lemon yellow
33 Bright golden yellow
34 Hot turquoise
35 Chinese blue
36 Clear teal
37 Emerald turquoise
38 True green
39 Emerald green
40 Pine
41 Periwinkle
42 Violet
43 Bright periwinkle
44 Purple
45 True blue
46 Medium blue
47 Royal blue
48 Navy

Wardrobe planning for your season

ON the following pages I have given, for each seasonal type, a suggested 12-piece wardrobe plan for working women. It is colour co-ordinated to help you create many different outfits. When putting your wardrobe together, aim to co-ordinate fabrics and styles, as well as colour, to make all pieces endlessly interchangeable.

Once you have built a fundamental working wardrobe you can begin adding other pieces to lend more excitement and even more possibilities.

CLEAR SPRING

Colour Combinations: Charcoal/Warm pink/Warm pastel pink/Purple

1. **Jacket:** Charcoal
2. **Jacket:** Warm pink
3. **Dress:** Purple
4. **Skirt:** Charcoal
5. **Skirt:** Warm pink
6. **Skirt:** Charcoal and Warm pink weave
7. **Trousers:** Charcoal
8. **Blouse:** Purple
9. **Blouse:** Warm pink and Charcoal
10. **Blouse:** Ivory
11. **Blouse:** Warm pastel pink
12. **Sweater:** Charcoal cardigan or swing wrap

WARM SPRING

Colour Combinations: Golden brown/Buttermilk/Rust/Yellow gold

1. **Jacket:** Golden brown
2. **Jacket:** Buttermilk
3. **Dress:** Rust
4. **Skirt:** Golden brown
5. **Skirt:** Buttermilk
6. **Skirt:** Golden brown/Rust/Buttermilk weave
7. **Trousers:** Golden brown
8. **Blouse:** Yellow gold
9. **Blouse:** Golden brown and Buttermilk
10. **Blouse:** Buttermilk and Rust
11. **Blouse:** Rust and Yellow gold
12. **Sweater:** Golden brown cardigan or swing wrap

LIGHT SPRING

Colour Combinations: Camel/Ivory/Clear aqua/Peach

1. **Jacket**: Ivory and Camel
2. **Jacket**: Camel
3. **Dress**: Ivory (long sleeve)
4. **Skirt**: Camel
5. **Skirt**: Ivory
6. **Skirt**: Camel and Ivory weave
7. **Trousers**: Camel
8. **Blouse**: Ivory
9. **Blouse**: Ivory and Clear aqua
10. **Blouse**: Clear aqua
11. **Blouse**: Peach and Aqua
12. **Sweater**: Ivory cardigan or swing wrap

LIGHT SUMMER

Colour Combinations: Light charcoal/Medium blue/Rose/Soft white

1. **Jacket**: Light charcoal
2. **Jacket**: Medium blue
3. **Dress**: Rose
4. **Skirt**: Light charcoal
5. **Skirt**: Medium blue
6. **Skirt**: Light charcoal/Medium blue/Soft white weave
7. **Trousers**: Light charcoal
8. **Blouse**: Soft white
9. **Blouse**: Soft white and Grey
10. **Blouse**: Medium blue and Soft white
11. **Blouse**: Medium blue and Rose
12. **Sweater**: Medium blue cardigan or swing wrap

COOL SUMMER

Colour Combinations: Blue charcoal Soft white/Raspberry/Icy pink

1. **Jacket**: Blue charcoal
2. **Jacket**: Soft white
3. **Dress**: Raspberry
4. **Skirt**: Charcoal blue-grey
5. **Skirt**: Soft white
6. **Skirt**: Blue charcoal and Soft white weave
7. **Trousers**: Blue charcoal
8. **Blouse**: Soft white
9. **Blouse**: Raspberry
10. **Blouse**: Raspberry, Blue charcoal and Soft white
11. **Blouse**: Icy pink
12. **Sweater**: Soft white cardigan/swing wrap

SOFT SUMMER

Colour Combinations: Pewter/Amethyst/Dusty rose/Soft white

1. **Jacket**: Pewter
2. **Jacket**: Amethyst
3. **Dress**: Dusty rose
4. **Skirt**: Pewter
5. **Skirt**: Amethyst
6. **Skirt**: Pewter/Amethyst/Soft white weave
7. **Trousers**: Pewter
8. **Blouse**: Dusty rose
9. **Blouse**: Soft white and Amethyst
10. **Blouse**: Pewter and Amethyst
11. **Blouse**: Pewter and Dusty rose
12. **Sweater**: Pewter cardigan or swing wrap

SOFT AUTUMN

Colour Combinations: Olive green/ Khaki/Bittersweet/Ivory

1. **Jacket**: Olive
2. **Jacket**: Khaki
3. **Dress**: Bittersweet
4. **Skirt**: Olive
5. **Skirt**: Khaki
6. **Skirt**: Olive/Khaki/Ivory weave
7. **Trousers**: Olive
8. **Blouse**: Ivory and Olive
9. **Blouse**: Bittersweet
10. **Blouse**: Bittersweet and Olive
11. **Blouse**: Ivory
12. **Sweater**: Olive cardigan or swing wrap

WARM AUTUMN

Colour Combinations: Golden brown/ Bronze/Light clear gold/Buff

1. **Jacket**: Golden brown
2. **Jacket**: Bronze
3. **Dress**: Light clear gold
4. **Skirt**: Golden brown
5. **Skirt**: Bronze
6. **Skirt**: Golden brown and Bronze weave
7. **Trousers**: Golden brown
8. **Blouse**: Light clear gold
9. **Blouse**: Bronze and Light clear gold
10. **Blouse**: Buff
11. **Blouse**: Bronze and Buff
12. **Sweater**: Bronze cardigan or swing wrap

DEEP AUTUMN

Colour Combinations: Black brown/ Rust/Ivory/Mariold

1. **Jacket**: Black brown
2. **Jacket**: Rust
3. **Dress**: Marigold
4. **Skirt**: Black brown
5. **Skirt**: Rust
6. **Skirt**: Black brown/Rust weave
7. **Trousers**: Black brown
8. **Blouse**: Rust and Ivory
9. **Blouse**: Rust and Marigold
10. **Blouse**: Ivory
11. **Blouse**: Marigold
12. **Sweater**: Black brown cardigan or swing wrap

DEEP WINTER

Colour Combinations: Black/Red/White/ Lemon yellow

1. **Jacket**: Black
2. **Jacket**: Red
3. **Dress**: Red
4. **Skirt**: Black
5. **Skirt**: Red
6. **Skirt**: Black/Red pattern, blend
7. **Trousers**: Black
8. **Blouse**: White
9. **Blouse**: Red/Lemon/White pattern
10. **Blouse**: Lemon
11. **Blouse**: Red and White
12. **Sweater**: White cardigan or swing wrap

COOL WINTER

Colour Combinations: Navy/Stone/Magenta

1. **Jacket:** Navy

2. **Jacket:** Stone

3. **Dress:** Magenta

4. **Skirt:** Navy

5. **Skirt:** Stone

6. **Skirt:** Navy and Stone weave/pattern

7. **Trousers:** Navy

8. **Blouse:** Magenta

9. **Blouse:** Magenta and Navy

10. **Blouse:** Navy and Stone

11. **Blouse:** Navy

12. **Sweater:** Navy cardigan or swing wrap

CLEAR WINTER

Colour Combinations: Charcoal/Royal blue/White/Icy blue

1. **Jacket:** Charcoal

2. **Jacket:** Royal blue

3. **Dress:** Royal blue

4. **Skirt:** Charcoal

5. **Skirt:** Royal blue

6. **Skirt:** Charcoal/Royal blue pattern, blend

7. **Trousers:** Charcoal

8. **Blouse:** White

9. **Blouse:** Icy blue

10. **Blouse:** Charcoal and Icy blue

11. **Blouse:** White and Royal blue

12. **Sweater:** White cardigan or swing wrap

Fabric guide

NATURAL FABRICS

Name	Description	Good For	Care Instructions
BROCADE	Rich woven fabric with raised pattern. Shiny or matt. Can be cotton, silk, viscose or mixture	Subtle treatments for scarves and blouses, or in more elaborate patterns and texture in dresses, jackets, etc	Dry clean
COTTON	Fibre from pods of cotton plant. Good for clothing because it's absorbent and allows air to circulate	Wide usage in fashion including underwear, blouses, dresses, jackets, skirts, sportswear and rainwear	Special finishes are used on most cotton to minimise care, such as to prevent shrinking, ease of pressing, maintaining pleats, etc. Usually washable by machine or hand

Types of Cotton

Name	Description	Good For	Care Instructions
Calico	Generic term for plain cotton. Strong yet loose weave	Summer and casual wear	Hand wash
Cambric	Lightweight, tightly woven cotton with a stiff, smooth finish	With crease resistant finish, good for dresses, shirts, suits	Hand wash
Cambray	Plain cotton with some dyed fibres giving a speckled effect. Quite durable	Sportswear, especially summertime	Hand or machine wash
Chintz	Cotton weave usually with a glazed finish	Best for interiors but also for summer dresses or jackets	Don't dry clean (you'll lose the glaze). Hand or gentle machine wash
Corduroy	Pile cotton of lengthwise cords	For sportswear, especially trousers, country shirts and skirts	Machine wash
Denim	A twill cotton pre-shrunk before use for strength. Very durable	Sportswear (especially for Naturals)	Machine wash

Name	Description	Good For	Care Instructions
Dotted Swiss	Fine, stiff cotton with a spotted effect	Delicate treatments in blouses, collars and dresses (very Romantic)	Hand wash
Flannelette	A cotton interpretation of wool flannel	Sleepwear	Machine wash
Gingham	Lightweight cotton woven in dyed yarns to form a check	Sports and casual wear as well as tablewear	Machine wash
Lawn	Lightweight cotton, sometimes blended with polyester	Blouses and hankies	Hand wash
Muslin	Often cotton, but also a generic term for soft, loose, open weaves. Good as a base for embroidered details	Blouses, summer dresses and skirts	Hand or machine wash on gentle cycle
Organdy	Lightweight plain cotton given a stiff finish	Blouses and dresses (evening only)	Hand wash
Oxford	Cotton woven with two yarns (often one white, one coloured). Gives a fresh, soft finish	Blouses, summer dresses	Machine wash
Percale	Good quality, tightly woven fabric often with glazed finish	Summer blouses, dresses and skirts	Machine wash
Sea Island	Best quality cotton from the West Indies	Its fine lustre makes it best in summer blouses, dresses and skirts	Machine wash
Seersucker	A woven cotton (often other fibres as well) producing alternating smooth and puckered surfaces usually in different coloured strips. Very durable	Jackets, skirts and blouses (summer weight only)	Machine wash
Sharkskin	Firm, tightly woven or knitted with a matt finish. Originally cotton but may be man made	Suits or crisp dresses	Dry clean
Velour	Heavy pile cotton fabric with a soft, velvet feel. (Other types of velour available.) Doesn't drape	Jackets, dresses, skirts	Machine wash. Note: Will soften with laundering
Voile	Hard spun yarns that create a light texture. See also Silk voile	Blouses, dresses	Gentle machine or hand wash
Whipcords	Twill lines that create a cord effect. Very durable	Jackets, skirts and trousers	Machine wash
DAMASK	Fabric with a woven pattern. May be cotton, linen, wool or silk	Aside from soft furnishings, damask comes in and out of fashion for jackets, blouses and dresses	Dry clean

Name	Description	Good For	Care Instructions
FOULARD	Refers to a printed fabric with an evenly repeated shiny pattern. Can be wool, silk or other fibres	Blouses, ties and scarves. Can be too much in large doses, so not suitable for dresses for work	Wash according to fibre. Check label
HOPSACK	A loose weave with the effect of a basket. Can be wool or cotton or mixed	Summer jackets. Skirts, blouses and trousers	Dry clean
LINEN	Spun from flax but too often made from viscose, polyester and other man-made fibres that are linen-like. Loose, thready appearance. Natural linen breathes and absorbs moisture	Excellent in spring and summer for casual and some business wear. For the latter choose linen blends with some man-made fibre or treatment to minimise wrinkles. The linen look is a very natural, crumpled effect	Handwash natural linen. Dry clean 'linen look' blends
SILK	Produced from caterpillars of the Bombyx and Antherea moths. Soft lustre and draping qualities make it an extensively used fabric	Fairly good crease shedding ability so good for blouses, dresses and scarves	Hand wash or dry clean. Check label
Types of Silk			
Silk crêpe	Silk fabric with crinkled or puckered effect. (Other types of crêpe available)	Blouses, evening or summer dresses	Hand wash
Silk crêpe de Chine	Refers to silk fabric with soft, blurred effect. (Other types of crêpe de Chine available)	Blouses, dresses, casual tops, trousers and skirts	Hand wash
Silk georgette	Sheer, lightweight silk with a crêpe effect. (Other types of georgette available)	Blouses, dresses, evening wear. Romantic as well as Dramatic, depending on style	Dry clean
Silk voile	Lightweight fabric in handspun silk with open texture. (Other types of voile available)	Casual wear, e.g. jackets and dresses. Very natural effect	Dry clean
WOOL	From sheep, lamb, goat, camel or llama fleece. Of variable characteristics and quality (merino the finest) with natural resilience and warm, soft properties.	Coats, suits, dresses, sweaters	Hand or gentle machine wash or dry clean. Check label. Fine wools are best stored folded rather than hung as they can stretch and loose their shape
Types of wool			
Alpaca	From the animal of the same name (llama family) with soft, fine hair. Not suitable for dyeing so used	Lightweight suitings and dresses	Hand wash or dry clean

Name	Description	Good For	Care Instructions
	in its natural colours of black, brown, camel or white		
Barathea	Pebbled hopsack wool available in medium and heavy weights. Hardwearing	Jackets and coats	Dry clean
Botany	A whole range of fabrics made from the finest merino wool	Suiting fabrics. Gives elegant appearance	Dry clean
Bouclé	Fabric woven from wool yarn looped at intervals giving a nubby texture. Also made from other fibres	Winter suits and sweaters. Can be used all over or as trimming. Softens the line of a garment	Dry clean
Camel hair	From the undercoat of the Bactrian camel. Unsuitable for dyeing so used in its beautiful natural 'camel' colour. Soft in texture, not as durable as wool	Coats, jackets and suits	Dry clean. Garments require rest between wearings
Cashgora	From a new cross bred goat. Its soft undercoat produces a warm, fine fibre	Mainly sweaters	Dry clean
Cashmere	Very fine undercoat of the Kashmir goat. Not very durable	Soft, warm and fine. Best for sweaters and shawls	Dry clean. Fold for storage in drawers rather than hang. Garments require rest between wearings
Cavalry twill	A firmly woven woollen cloth	Trousers, menswear and raincoats	Dry clean
Cloqué	Knitted woollen fabric with bubbled effect from knitting extra loops	Sweaters, casual dresses	Dry clean or hand wash with care
Flannel	A plain woollen weave that feels soft and warm due to its textured finish. Very durable and hardwearing	Wintertime jackets and suits	Requires pressing with regular wear. Dry clean
Gabardine	Tightly woven worsted wool with fine lines in the fabric. Can be combined with cotton or other fibres. Hard wearing	Elegant suits, coats and trousers. Excellent investment for your best work suit	Dry clean
Herringbone	Woollen weaves with the effect of a 'z' or 's' in the fabric. Hard wearing	Coats, jackets and skirts. More casual or country than business	Dry clean
Lambswool	The fleece of baby lambs. Very soft	Sweaters, blouses and simple dresses	Dry clean or hand wash with care
Mohair	The long springy hair of the Angora goat. Very strong. Often woven with other fibres. Pure mohair can produce the finest	Suiting mainly	Dry clean

Name	Description	Good For	Care Instructions
	lightweight, albeit expensive, suiting. Retains a crisp finish		
Tweed	Originating in Scotland as a rough wool weave. Now also made from other fibres	Coats, jackets, trousers and suits. Finest tweeds possible for working suits but better for country and casual wear	Dry clean woollen tweeds. For others wash according to fibre
Wool crêpe	Loosely woven wool	Jackets, skirts, trousers and suits. Creates a softer look in business suits. Available in light (for summer) and medium weight (for winter)	Dry clean

MAN-MADE FABRICS

Name	Description	Good For	Care Instructions
ACRYLIC	A petroleum derivative yarn that has a soft feel and is relatively crease resistant. Can be very finely woven or produce nubby, wool-like effects. As with other manufactured fibres it does not breathe or provide the warmth of wool. Often blended with wool	Knitwear	Easy. Hand or machine wash
BLENDS	Polyester combined with a natural fabric, e.g. 60% wool, 40% polyester. Blended to minimise care and retain shape. The more polyester the less moisture absorption and comfort	Skirts, trousers, raincoats and blouses	Easy. Hand or machine wash. Often drip-dry. Check label
NYLON	A derivative of coke and tar spun for its strength and elasticity. High concentrated nylon fabrics cling, don't 'breathe' and are prone to static	Tights and sportswear	Easy. Hand or machine wash
POLYESTER	Comes from petroleum and used extensively in clothing. Can be processed to look and feel like silk or cotton. Varying quality at every price level	Used in everything but tights	Easy. Hand or machine wash
VISCOSE	Not totally man-made as viscose is a derivative of wood pulp manufactured into a fibre. Usually treated to make crease-resistant	Blouses, dresses and casual wear	Some finishes are adversely affected by laundering so read care label. Dry cleaning is safest

Bibliography and further reading

BODY LANGUAGE

Body Language by Jane Lyle (Hamlyn 1990)
Body Language by Allan Pease (Sheldon Press 1981)
Manwatching by Desmond Morris (Granada 1978)
Silent Language by George Patounas (Allied Training Inc. 1986)
Your Total Image by Philippa Davies (Piatkus 1990)

COLOUR

A Color Notation by A. H. Munsell (Mácbeth, Kollmorgen 1981)
Colour Me Beautiful by Carole Jackson (Piatkus 1983)
Healing through Colour by Theo Gimbel (CW Daniel Press 1987)
Know Yourself Through Colour by Marie Louise Lacy (Aquarian Press 1989)
The Luscher Colour Test by Dr. Max Luscher (Washington Square Press 1969)

FABRICS

The Encyclopedia of Fashion Details by Patrick Ireland, (B. T. Batsford 1987)
Technology of Textile Properties by Marjorie Taylor (Forbes Publications 1990)

FACIAL FITNESS

Eva Fraser's Facial Workout by Eva Fraser (Viking 1991)
Joseph Corvo's Zone Therapy by Joseph Corvo (Century 1990)

HEALTH & FITNESS

Beautiful Body, Beautiful Skin by Norma Knox (Piatkus 1990)
Holistix by Carole Caplin (Sidgwick & Jackson 1990)
Perfect Health by Deepak Chopra MD (Bantam 1990)
Ultra Health by Leslie Kenton (Ebury Press 1989)

INTERNATIONAL IMAGE/ETIQUETTE

The Complete Book of Business Etiquette Lynne Brennan and David Block (Piatkus 1991)
Guide des Bonnes Mannières et du Protocole en Europe by Jacques Gandouin (Pergamon Books, Fixot 1989)
Handbook for Women Travellers by Maggie and Gemma Moss (Piatkus 1987)
Mind Your Manners by John Mole (The Industrial Society 1990)
The International Businesswoman by Marlene Rossman (Praegar 1986)
The World Class Executive by Neil Chesanow (Rowson Associates, NY 1985)

MAKE-UP

Colour Me Beautiful Make-Up Book by Carole Jackson (Piatkus 1987)
8 Minute Make-Overs by Claire Miller (Acropolis Books 1984)
Face to Face with Barbara Daly A Make-Up Lesson on Video (The Body Shop 1990)

STYLE

Always In Style by Doris Pooser (Piatkus 1986)
Clothes Sense by Jane Procter (Doubleday 1985)
The Language of Clothes by Allison Lurie (Heinemann 1982)
Vogue Pattern Magazines by subscription or via fabric pattern stores

SUCCESSFUL DRESSING

The Professional Image by Susan Bixler (Putnam 1984)
Wardrobe: Develop your style and confidence by Susie Faux with Philippa Davies (Piatkus 1988)
Your Public Best by Lillian Brown (Newmarket Press 1989)
Presenting Yourself: A personal image guide for women by Mary Spillane (Piatkus 1993)

WOMEN'S DEVELOPMENT

A Woman In Your Own Right by Anne Dickson (Quartet Books 1982)
Making The Most of Yourself by Gill Cox and Sheila Danow (Sheldon Press 1989)
Megatrends 2000 by John Naisbett and Patricia Aburdene (Sidgwick & Jackson 1982)
Passages by Gail Sheehy (Bantam Books 1976)
Pathfinders by Gail Sheehy (Bantam Books 1981)
Springboard by Liz Willis and Jenny Daisley (Hawthorn Press 1990)
The Beauty Myth by Naomi Wolf (Chatto & Windus 1990)
The Influential Woman by Lee Bryce (Piatkus 1989)
Unfinished Business by Maggie Scarf (Doubleday 1980)
Your Total Image: How to communicate success by Philippa Davies (Piatkus 1990)

Index

Page numbers in *italic* refer to the illustrations

More from COLOR ME BEAUTIFUL

• Personal Image Classes

Color Me Beautiful have a comprehensive network of highly trained image consultants who offer individual and group consultations on colour, style and make-up. You can visit a consultant for a one-to-one session or bring a friend for a joint session. Each consultation includes a workbook and at our popular colour analysis session you receive an elegant wallet with 48 fabric swatches representing your best colours.

• Color Me Beautiful Products

An exclusive range of cosmetics, skincare, scarves and fashion accessories are available from your local CMB consultant or direct via our mail-order catalogue.

• A Color Me Beautiful Career

If you enjoy helping people make the most of themselves, CMB can offer a challenging and rewarding career. Call or send for details and you will receive a free career pack on how to become a CMB Image Consultant. This flexible career can be run on a full or part-time basis, from a business premises or your home and can offer an exciting add-on service alongside an existing, compatible business.

• Business Seminars and Promotions

Entertaining and informative presentations and seminars are in demand by retailers as well as companies who recognise the importance of a good personal and company image. CMB have developed exciting joint promotions and valued incentives for clients who want loyal customers or staff to feel recognised and rewarded.

For futher details on any of the above services/products, please complete and return the freepost information request form below. Alternatively, call us on 0171- 627 5211

INFORMATION REQUEST FORM

Please send me information on the following:

(tick the boxes as necessary)

Personal Image Classes ☐

CMB Products ☐

CMB Career ☐

Business Seminars ☐

NAME: _____ *(please print)*

ADDRESS: _____

_____

_____

DAYTIME TELEPHONE NO: _____

SG

POSTAGE
PAID

CMB Image Consultants
FREEPOST
London SW8 3BR